also by Daniel Stih

I0130046

Dust Money: How to Clean Your Home and
Belongings After Mold Remediation So You Don't
Have to Throw Everything Away

Rent Money: The Toxic Mold Handbook for
Tenants and Landlords

Mold Money

How to Save Thousands of Dollars on Mold Remediation and Make Sure the Mold is Gone

Healthy Living Spaces
369 Montezuma Ave #169
Santa Fe, NM 87501

DISCLAIMER

Every building has a set of circumstances that is unique for which additional specifications or modifications of the information presented here may be required. If everything you need to know were covered, here it would be a more technical read. The intent is to provide basic information that you can use to make informed decisions. The author does not assume responsibility for actions you take based on reading this book. If you want specific recommendations please call Healthy Living Spaces (505) 603-8101. We will take responsibility for everything we tell you.

Unconditional Release of Liability

You hereby release and exempt the author and Healthy Living Spaces LLC from any and all liability and responsibility regarding the use of any of the information contained here.

ACKNOWLEDGEMENTS

Special thanks to Will Spates at Indoor Environmental Technologies in Clearwater, Florida. Will was an early mentor of mine. He always shared what he knew generously and with enthusiasm for his work.

TABLE OF CONTENTS

EMERGENCY MOLD PREVENTION

How to Prevent Mold From Growing

We'll get to the basics in a moment. If a water leak has just occurred, it's imperative to dry things out as quickly as possible. Other than water, mold requires time to grow. This may be as little as three days to a week, depending on the amount of water and types of mold.

Call your insurance company.

Do not wait for your insurance company to call you back. Look in the phone book or on the Internet for Water Damage Restoration Company and call them immediately.

A few issues to be aware of:

The drying company will want to dry things out as quick as possible to avoid mold growing; the adjuster and your insurance company will want to save money.

Your insurance company may recommend a company to you but you don't have to use them. You should pick the best drying company you can find. Your insurance has to cover you if they cover the loss. Don't confuse water damage with mold coverage. For dry-out, policyholders are covered for the structural amount, i.e. $400,000 if that's the value of your house. Mold is not what we are talking about (yet).

It is best to wait for the adjuster to come. If the adjuster can't come for a few days, you and the drying company should ask your insurance company what you should do to prevent mold from growing. Talk to a supervisor. A homeowner may want to tell the drying company to do what ever is necessary to dry things and prevent mold from growing and assume the risk, regardless if insurance will pay or not.

There is a company running drying jobs on behalf of many insurance companies. They are the middlemen that insurance companies use to save money. This company has their own adjusters who communicate with drying companies instead of the drying companies communicating directly with insurance companies. This company guarantees the insurance companies that the drying will take only three days. Where did three days come from? They claim some references say that every building material can be dry in three days. In fact the reference says building materials *must* be dry in three days; otherwise mold can grow. Some drying companies may refuse to work under the intention to save money instead of getting things dried the quickest way possible.

For example, if you have a tile floor on top of a wood subfloor, some of the tile may need to be removed. The adjuster may require the drying company to try and dry it with fans. The drying company may tell the adjuster they need to remove some of the flooring. The adjuster may start fighting with the drying company and not approve what the drying company wants to do.

If the adjuster does not want to do what the drying company recommends, tell the drying company to contact a supervisor at your insurance. Your insurance may say, "Ok, remove part of the floor." This is usually limited to when the drying company, not the homeowner, makes the call. Make sure you have a drying company who knows what they are doing. Use common sense. If it doesn't seem like what is being done will dry things in three days, it probably won't.

If the adjuster and your insurance decide they don't want to follow the drying company's recommendations, the drying company may write your insurance an email that says, "Per our conversation...I alerted you to the possibility that mold might grow if we don't_____. Your decision was to wait and send out an adjuster in x number of days. I therefore decline any responsibility and all liability with respect to mold growing." In these types of circumstances you should write your insurance a similar email.

Why do adjusters make it difficult? It's the same with any business. If an adjuster does ten jobs for insurance X, insurance X is going to ask them to save them some money.

.

Introduction

I've had a microscope since I was twelve. In 1978, my brothers and I opened Sun Laboratorys (we spelled Laboratories wrong) in the utility room of our parents home. I let milk spoil and examined what grew under a microscope. Wanting us to be safe, my mom made us walk to the university and talk to professors who sent us home with beakers, flasks, microscope slides and other supplies.

Moving forward, I got a degree in Aerospace Engineering and worked at Motorola in Phoenix for eleven years. One

THE **ROADRUNNER**

MOTOROLA INC.
Semiconductor Group

A MOTOROLA WEEKLY PERSONNEL DEPARTMENT PUBLICATION
APRIL 12, 1979

EAGER SCIENTISTS
TAKE OVER LAUNDRY ROOM

52nd Street - Judy Stih, Regional Trainer in Sales Support for John Moran, noticed her 3 boys were playing in the laundry room but really hadn't paid that much attention to the activities until the boys asked her to look over their Civilian Report No. 001. The report showed recordings and drawings of experiments they had been performing in their laboratory (the laundry room).

Deciding the eager young scientists should be aware of chemical safety precautions, she sent them to ASU for help. The boys were given sound safety advice on the correct use of safety equipment when working with chemicals.

The boys first became interested in scientific experimenting while living in Mentor, Ohio. One day they visited a Flea Market with their grandmother and purchased a chemistry set and a biology set for $1.50 each. These purchases have led them to such experiments as: dissecting, identifying and labeling the parts of frogs and grasshoppers by biologist,

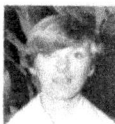

Danny, 12 years old; to identifying rocks and minerals by geologist, Todd, 10 years old; to producing oxygen from combining Hydrogen Peroxide with Magnesium Dioxide by Chemist, John, 14 years old.

The laboratory boasts microscopes, labeled drawings, flasks, newsarticles on the sciences, air-tight plastic chemical bottles, preserved frogs and starfish, and a small scientific library...all kept in very neat order. "We clean each day," said John.

The ambitious boys prefer working in their lab rather than participating in other activities. They are currently working on Civilian Report No. 002 which has a projected due date of June, 1979.

Donations of old science books and textbooks would be appreciated by the young scientists. They are quickly outgrowing their small library. If you don't want that old Chemistry textbook, give their mother a call at 244-3902.

Shown posing before their laboratory are (L. to R.): John, Danny, and Todd Stih.

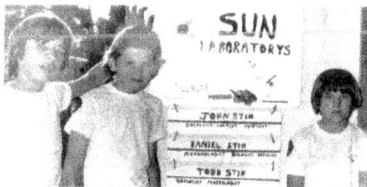

Sharer of the laundry room and mother of the aspiring young scientists is Judy Stih (Left Photo).

SUN
LABORATORYS

Sun Laboratorys, circa 1978.

day, tired of the heat and of being an engineer for a large corporation, I quit my job and moved to a small town where as fate would have it - I ended up working as a handyman.

I had so much work I didn't know what to do with it all. Then one day, I started to get sick and was tired all the time. At first I blamed it on working too much. Then I found out it was from the hazardous stuff I was being exposed to. The work I was doing, the homes I was going into - that's what was making me sick.

Once I was aware of that, I began to realize there are a lot of people out there who are sick because of their homes. If was happening to me, it had to be happening to them. So I decided to find ways of getting rid of what was making us sick. Through my research, inspecting and testing thousands of homes and offices, I found that the cause of many people's illness is mold.

I have lectured and been interviewed on over one hundred radio and television stations. In addition to other certifications, I am a Council-Certified Microbial Consultant and Council-Certified Indoor Environmental Consultant, Board-awarded by the American Council for Accredited Certification (ACAC). I've taken all the courses but like most things in life, there is no substitute for experience. My grandmother's house was my first mold remediation job.

Nana wasn't feeling good. She bought the equipment I needed to remove the mold from her house: HEPA air scrubber and HEPA vacuum cleaner. Nothing but plain soap and water in those days. Why do people think they need to use chemicals to remove mold these days? So many professionals, those you count on to do an honest and effective job, use chemicals to treat mold instead of remove it. They should know better. Do they?

I wrote this book because I am disappointed with how the industry has developed. When I learned how to remediate mold it was quite clear that bleach is not the answer – that, as you will learn, plain soap and water are *more* effective than bleach. As contractors jumped on the bandwagon to make money, they have either been taught wrong or have been convinced into buying products to treat mold. They have forgotten or did not learn the basics. Some mold remediators do not know how to use their equipment the right way but charge you high dollar by the day for using it.

I am going to tell you how mold is supposed to be removed and why you are paying too much for mold remediation.

I am going to tell you how you can save money *and* make sure the mold is removed instead of covered by sealants, antimicrobials and other gimmicks. If any contractor tells you that my advice is too difficult to follow or will cost you more to follow - ask them which part and why. I guarantee you will not receive an intelligent answer.

The bigger the remediation company, the bigger the rip offs. If they say they do government work, beware.

Please send me your comments. Contact me through, www.HealthyLivingSpaces.com. I am available for phone consultations, travel and expert witness testimony.

Part 1: Mold 101

DEBUNKING MYTHS AND DIS-INFORMATION

Chapter 1

Mold Basics

What Mold Remediators Don't Want You to Know

First I want to give my regards to the good mold remediators out there. You know who you are. You earn your money honestly by doing quality work.

Now that I've cleared the air, here's what those doing mold remediation the wrong way, don't want you to know. What they are doing is not that difficult. They make lots of money charging you what a good mold remediator does (remove mold) and they don't remove the mold or all of it. Many charge for equipment they do not know how to use, equipment that might as well not be used, and equipment that could be contaminating your house with mold from the last job it was used it on.

The average remediator does not want you to know this - they are doing the same thing a general contractor can do: tear out drywall and make a big mess. A good mold remediator ALSO does an impeccable job of cleaning. It's time consuming. That's not the norm. The norm is, let's charge a lot of money because it's "mold", then get in there and tear things out while the owner thinks we are doing some kind of specialized, technical work.

Some remediators scare you to the point you can't pause to ask yourself, "Is it that bad? Do I have to do this?" You're like a deer in the headlights panicking for the safety of your family. You may feel like just writing them a check. The trouble is, "Just getting it done," doesn't mean it will be done right. Sometimes remediators make things worse.

I've worked in various states across the country and it's the same wherever I go - good intentions by mold remediators that do not understand how mold is supposed to be removed. I find companies that complain about how difficult (more expensive) it will be to remove mold after I explain how it's supposed to be done.

Most states do not have mold laws. Laws aren't the answer. All the remediator has to do is pay a fee and they get certified.

What Some Mold Remediators Don't Know

Here's an estimate from a remediation company that also did the testing:

"After inspecting the property, test results show elevated counts of *Aspergillus/Penicillin* mold."

(Yes, this is a direct quote. It says Penicillin, a type of antibiotic, instead of *Penicillium*, a type of mold).

"The following remediation needs to be done to bring down the level of microbial contamination: Mold eradication by fogging and sanitization using a sanitizer/odor machine."

What is wrong with this? First, fogging and sanitizers do not remove mold. I believe the mold remediator does not know this. He might not want to because he makes money off using them. Perhaps he believes the mold is treated, if so, he should indicate that. Instead, he presents it as if the mold will be removed. This estimate uses the word, "eradicated".

Sanitizing will do nothing to bring down the level of contamination as he suggests. Testing will still detect the mold. It will still be there.

Myth - Only Certain Types of Mold are Toxic

It's a hostile world for mold. Other molds want to grow, bacteria multiply like rabbits around you and some insects want to eat you. Molds produce toxins to protect themselves. Every mold has a list of toxins it can create. The toxins differ depending on what the mold is competing with.

There are 250,000 different species of molds. Of the molds that have been studied, each is capable of producing a dozen or more toxins. *Cladosporium* for example, the most common outdoor mold, is used to produce Cladosporin, an antifungal metabolite used in athlete's foot treatment. (The synthetic version is Asperentin.)

Mold does not produce toxins all of the time. It takes energy to make toxins. If you grow mold in a petri dish in the laboratory by itself, it will not produce toxins. If it doesn't need to expend the energy, it won't.

Testing for mycotoxins is rarely done in a building. The tests are expensive and you have to test for all the possible toxins that all the molds are known to be capable of producing. What if you miss some? Laboratories test for only three or four.

To keep it simple, no professional should be giving you advice based on the *type* of mold present. The standards for mold remediation are the same regardless of the types of mold present.

Black Mold

When people say "black" mold they are referring to *Stachybotrys*. *Stachybotrys* is not the only mold that can be black. There are three primary colors, a quarter million species of mold. The same type of mold can be different colors. The front of a mold culture is often a different color than the back. Molds change color with age. *Penicillium chrysogenum*, the organism that produces penicillin, forms colonies that are initially white but turn blue-green with age. *Aspergillus niger* produces a white mycelium before turning yellow and forming black spores. *Cladosporium* can be black. These are a few examples.

It's More Than Mold

Some ask, "If outdoor mold can't hurt me why should I be worried about indoor mold?"

The answer is simple - mold growth doesn't belong indoors. Since you can remove it, why wouldn't you? The answer is also complex.

Mold did not grow because it liked the color of the carpet. It grew because there was a source of water. With water came other microorganisms. There is a long list of allergens and irritants due to microorganisms that thrive in damp conditions. Mold is the tip of the iceberg. Some might make you sick, some not. In terms of testing, mold is the easiest: Eventually, you *see* mold growing.

According to the Institute of Medicine of the National Academies, the other factors responsible for health effects associated with dampness include: bacteria, allergens of microbial origin, structural components of fungal spores (glucans), structural components of bacterial cells (endotoxins), metabolite by-products including microbial volatile organic compounds (mVOCs), mycotoxins, allergens and pathogens from cockroaches, ants, termites and other insects. Release of these components vary, depending on the environmental factors. Dampness can also damage building materials causing or exacerbating the release of chemicals and non-biological particles. Because it is impractical to evaluate a building and it's occupants for exposure to each and all of these components, the general recommendation is to remove water damaged materials vs. attempting to quantify the significance of any mold that may or may not be present.

What if the mold is dead?

How do you tell if mold is dead? A mold spore is like a seed. How do you tell if a seed is dead until you water it to try to grow a plant?

How does mold die? Mold can go into a resting stage. It might look dead - it's dormant. Gardeners call it over-wintering.

Some say sunlight and UV light neutralize mold. If that were so, one would have allergies. Sunlight would have neutralized all the pollen and mold in the universe.

Does it matter? A pollen spore is allergenic regardless of its viability. It is similar with mold. All mold is allergenic, even the dead (non-viable) spores. All molds have the potential to be toxigenic. Toxins don't die.

In some ways dry mold may result in more of an exposure to mold than wet mold. Wet mold is sticky and does not become airborne as easy. As mold dries it desiccates into small pieces, becomes air-borne with the gentlest of disturbances, and may pass deeper into your lungs when you breathe the smaller particles. You might test for mold and think you don't have any because the dead stuff fragmented into gazillions of nano-sized particles that no laboratory can detect. Meanwhile you have symptoms.

Just remove the mold and save yourself from wondering.

Can I just Spray it with Bleach?

You can. Why would you? It would take a lot of bleach, a long contact time, you won't kill all the mold and the dead mold will still be there, as allergenic and as toxigenic as before.

The Neighbors did *This*

The company the neighbors hired for mold remediation may have treated the mold instead of removed it. Your neighbor might not care or want to know that there is still mold in their home. They probably paid a lot of money for mold remediation.

The next buyer or renter may be concerned that mold was treated instead of removed. If you sell your house and do not disclose that the mold was treated instead of removed, you are not disclosing there is mold.

Sound troublesome? It is. If you're paying to have mold removed, make sure it is removed instead of treated.

I Don't Have Symptoms

Some people wonder, "Will I get sick if I don't remove the mold?"

How people become sick from mold is partially still a mystery. Mold does not infect you like a disease. Infection is usually limited to people who are, for example, in the hospital, cut open for surgery.

Mycotoxins are substances on the cell walls of the spores and mycelium (roots of mold). You may be poisoned by a substance mold slathers itself with to protect it from other organisms. It enters in your blood stream when you breathe particles of mold or your skin comes in contact with them.

I am not a doctor; it's my opinion – I don't think mycotoxins are what make most people sick from mold. If you test a house for mycotoxins you have to collect a lot of dust for the lab to detect it. More commonly, eating food that has mold causes people (and animals) to become sick.

My experience is that only a few people out of a group will have allergies to mold. If I'm inspecting an office and everyone is having allergies, it's often not because of mold.

There are health problems related to long-term exposure to mold including neurologic disorders such as foggy thinking and organ damage. There are synergistic effects. A smoker may have a greater chance of having a reaction to mold than a non-smoker.

If you don't have symptoms consider yourself lucky. Don't gamble with your health – get the mold removed or get out.

If and how people are affected from mold varies by individual, their sensitivity, how compromised the immune system is, and a long list of factors that make assessing the potential risk to mold a risky endeavor. Just get rid of the mold.

Mold *growth* is not everywhere

Mold spores are everywhere. Mold *growth* is not everywhere. If you look under a microscope, you can find a mold spore in the dust of your home. Unless you have mold growing in your house, it will be a mushroom or common outdoor mold type. It's like finding a few spores of pollen in the dust. You'll find those too. (Unfortunate for those allergic to pollen.)

Unless you water them, the seeds made from pollen will not grow into plants in your living room. Similarly, unless you water them, the mold spores will not grow into a mold infestation in your house.

There are those who dismiss the idea that mold growing in homes is a problem. They can't see the justification for spending money to remove mold because it's "everywhere". Mold *growth* is not everywhere and does not belong in your home.

Will Insurance Pay?

Some do. Some don't. Most insurance companies cap mold coverage at $5,000. Where did that number come from? Good question. Insurance companies know the right thing is for them to cover mold. They are trying to cut their losses. If they throw you a bone they hope you will leave them alone.

Whether your insurance covers mold depends on the source of water and when it occurred. Typically there needs to be a sudden incident: roof leaks from a hailstorm, a dishwasher, washing machine or toilet hose exploding. The key word is *sudden*. Insurance will usually not pay for mold that slowly started to grow years ago and was recently discovered.

When Insurance Companies are to Blame

Sometimes your insurance is responsible for the mold that grew but will tell you, "Sorry, we don't cover mold." It's like getting in a car accident with your adjuster, an accident that is his fault and he tells you you're not covered. Why do you need coverage?

Case in point, an elderly woman had a roof leak. She called her home insurance. The insurance company waited ten days before sending out a drying company. The drying company found a small area with rot (mold) in the ceiling, called the insurance company and said, "We found mold." The insurance company told the drying company, "We don't cover mold. Get out of there."

The drying company left, leaving the wall in her bedroom cut open and a big, wet mess. They did not ask her if she wanted to dry things out anyway.

Mold grew where the new leak occurred.

The insurance adjuster told the woman, "Just spray it with bleach."

After an investigation by independent parties it was concluded if the insurance company had not told the drying company to leave, the majority of the mold would not have grown. The insurance did the right thing and paid to clean up the mess.

Insurance adjusters are not mold inspectors. When in doubt, they should request an assessment by a certified mold inspector. This should be part of the claim, paid the same way insurance companies pay adjusters and structural engineers. It should not come out of the deductible. If your insurance company tells you they won't pay for a mold inspection, what they are saying is that they are confident in their own assessment and do not need an expert's opinion. They assume responsibility for their actions.

What ever your insurance company tells you, ask them to put it in writing. Tell them you are recording the conversations you have with them.

Do I need to move out?

One of the reasons mold remediation is expensive are the engineering controls: air scrubbers, negative air pressure, containment, and so forth. This is to prevent mold from getting into the rest of your house during remediation activities that generate lots of dust such as removing walls and wire brushing and sanding. If the containment is set up the correct way you can live in your house while the work is being done. It might be noisy. Air scrubbers have big, loud fan motors inside them. The issue is a lot of remediators do not create the containment and install the air scrubbers the correct way. We'll get to that.

Interim Solutions

If you have decided on a course of action and are in the process of getting estimates to have the mold removed, there are some things you can do in the meantime to minimize exposure.

One is to buy a good air purifier. The IQAir Health Pro Plus is the only one I recommend based on testing it with a laser particle counter. Zero particles come out the exhaust. It's better than HEPA. Beware of air purifiers that say you don't need to change filters. Beware of air cleaners that use ozone or UV light. These don't work.

If there is mold in the furnace, air conditioning or duct-work - shut them off.

If mold is visible on a wall, consider carefully covering it with plastic and duct tape. Although this won't prevent all the spores from coming out, it might give you peace of mind. Be very careful covering mold. Mold spores are like dandelion spores in the wind waiting to disperse with the gentlest of agitation. I sometimes use clear, sticky carpet protector that comes in a roll and apply it to the part of the wall with mold visible.

An air scrubber set up to create a negative air pressure in the room is the only way to effectively isolate an area with mold. Place the air scrubber in the room with mold. Place the exhaust duct out the window and close the door. Now the air scrubber is acting as what is called a negative air machine. A negative (lower) air pressure is created in the room relative to the rest of the house. Air from the rest of the house will be pulled into the room. Air inside the room will be exhausted outdoors. This is called containment. You might consider buying an air scrubber and selling it on e-bay when you are finished. Suggestions are in the resource section of *Chapter 10: Consider Doing It Yourself.*

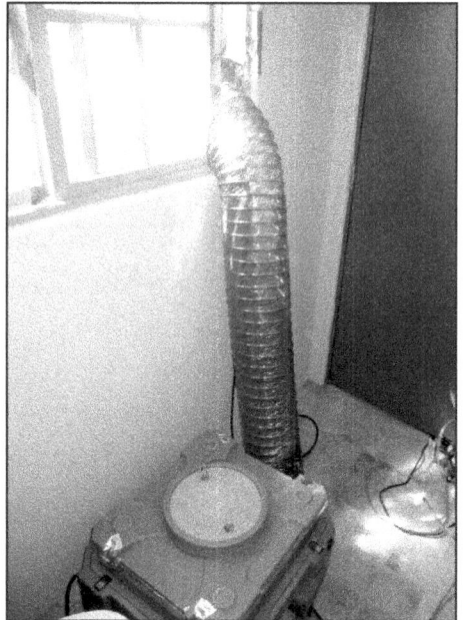

Air scrubber exhausted out a window.

Key Points To Remember From Chapter I

• Don't try to kill mold. Mold has a tough shell. It's made with chitin, the main component of exoskeletons of arthropods. "Dead" mold is still allergenic and potentially toxigenic.

• Mold can be removed the old fashioned way - hard work instead of chemicals. That's why mold remediation was traditionally expensive.

• It doesn't matter what kind of mold it is. Get rid of it all. Do not waste your time and money doing a science experiment.

• Sometimes your insurance is to blame. If your insurance company gives you advice remind them that they are assuming responsibility for giving it. Speak in an intelligent manner. If they say, "Just spray it with bleach," ask, "Are you familiar with the *S520 Standard for Professional Mold Remediation?* What page are you referencing?" Hire an attorney.

Chapter 2

Testing for Mold

You can't see mold

According to Chin S. Yang, Ph.D., a pioneer in microbiology testing, you can't see mold until there are at least one million spores per square inch of surface.

Cutting holes to look for mold can be misleading.

Cutting holes to look for mold can contaminate your house with mold. If mold is present, it's growing on the backside of the wall with spores hanging on, waiting for the gentlest of disturbances to knock them loose.

If a mold inspector says he has to cut a hole to look for mold ask him to leave. There are better ways to test for mold.

If you *see* mold, you don't need to test it

If you see mold you don't need to know what type it is. You have to have it removed. You do not need a mold inspector to test it. You need mold inspector to give you advice on how to remove it.

Self-test kits – Don't bother

You might think you can save money by doing your own testing and buy a self-test kit. You set test dishes out for a few hours, put the lids on, and ship them off to a laboratory. The laboratory tells you what kind and how many colonies of mold grew.

What's wrong with this?

I can't tell you how many times people call saying they have mold in their home, asking what they should do. I ask them how they know they have mold. They say they have x number of *Aspergillus/Penicillium* colonies in their test results, more than what is considered normal.

What grows in a petri dish does not translate to what, if any, mold is growing in your home. The agar is designed to grow mold. Somewhere in your house there is a spore that floated in from the outdoors. It takes only a single spore to grow into a million spores. It's similar to leaving a loaf of bread or piece of fruit on the kitchen table. Mold will grow on it. Does that mean there is mold in your house? Of course not.

The opposite happens too. There *is* mold in a house but the test grows only a few colonies, a level below which the lab considers there to be mold in the house. You might not think you have mold. You do. Why is this?

Dead mold, while still allergenic and potentially toxigenic, won't grow.

Not all types of mold like the same food. The company selling the test has to choose an agar preferred by most types of mold. There are 250,000 different species of mold. Which one did they pick? – An agar that supports most types of mold.

The agar in self-test kits does not support *Stachybotrys*. *Stachybotrys* is a slow grower. The test dish may become overgrown with common molds before *Stachybotrys* has a chance. There is a special agar used to culture *Stachybotrys*. If it were sold in stores you would need two tests - one that supports *Stachybotrys*, the other for the other types of mold. What about molds that prefer neither of these types of agars? Where does it end?

If it seems too good to be true it is. If you're trying to find the cheapest way to test for mold you are not going to obtain reliable results.

The 42-page laboratory report - What does it mean?

Not much.

Laboratories think they are perceived as better if they provide longer reports. The labs are reacting to their clients. Some inspectors think you will believe they did a better job if their reports are longer. How many charts, graphs and fugal glossaries do we need?

In one report I was asked to review, only one air sample was collected; only one type of mold was detected by the lab. The lab report was forty-two pages. The lab dedicated one page to each of twenty other types of molds, molds that were not detected. They included references, charts, graphs and links to information about mold. It appeared they were trying to educate the client about mold. What are you paying for when you have your house tested for mold? I suspect you want to know:

1 Is there mold?

2 Where?

That will not be in the lab report. It's your mold inspector's job to know where and how to test for mold and how to interpret the lab results.

If you find yourself confused by lengthy lab reports, don't take it personally. I leaf through to find the important stuff. If you have a good mold inspector they will write their own report that includes a narrative of what the results mean and where the mold is. They should not just hand you a lab report.

How to find a good mold inspector

Go to ACAC.org, the website for the American Council for Accredited Certification (ACAC).

Type your zip code in.

Look for a Certified Microbial Consultant, CMC.

Don't Google CMC. The ACAC was unsuccessful in trademarking the letters CMC. Many using them are not certified by the ACAC. Some on-line training companies sell the acronym for a fee.

The ACAC is accredited by the Engineering Standards Board. In addition to passing a test, those holding certifications have their field experience verified. Eight years of experience is required. They call whom you did work for eight years ago. While there is a chance someone has been doing it wrong for eight years, this is not typical with those certified by ACAC.

Ask about insurance. Most states do not have laws that require mold inspectors and remediators to have special insurance. In addition to General Liability, mold inspectors should have Environmental Consultants' Professional Liability Insurance. Mold remediators should have Pollution Liability Insurance. Some will tell you they have insurance. (Just like they say they are certified.) What they mean is, they have general liability insurance. Ask to see the policy.

Beware of Industrial Hygienists (IH's) claiming they don't need to be certified mold inspectors because they are Industrial Hygienists. They may not have the training or field experience that is required to be a certified microbial consultant. They should stick to testing factories where they assess workers for exposure to chemicals.

If the same company doing remediation says they will do the testing - walk away from using them for either. It's unethical to do both unless you live in a remote part of Alaska. Later I shall go into detail about a mold estimate that was from the same company that did the testing. This company gave the homeowner a $3,500 estimate to fog their home but could not say *where* the mold was and offered no guarantee.

Spend your money on a good mold inspector the first time. Don't shop for the cheapest, because typically those inspectors test a house and when the results show it has mold, they can't tell the client *where* the mold is.

Testing for Hidden Mold

I use a method called the Wall-Chek™. If performed correctly it's very effective at determining where mold is hiding. A small, pencil-size hole is drilled into a wall or ceiling. A tube is inserted, the air sucked out and sent to a laboratory. It's very sensitive. Unlike air samples that are collected in the middle of the room and may not detect mold that is present, with the Wall-Chek™ there are no false results.

Collecting a wall cavity sample is a specialized skill. Some mold inspectors do not like the test because they get false results. I had the opportunity to learn from Charlie Wiles, the man who invented it.

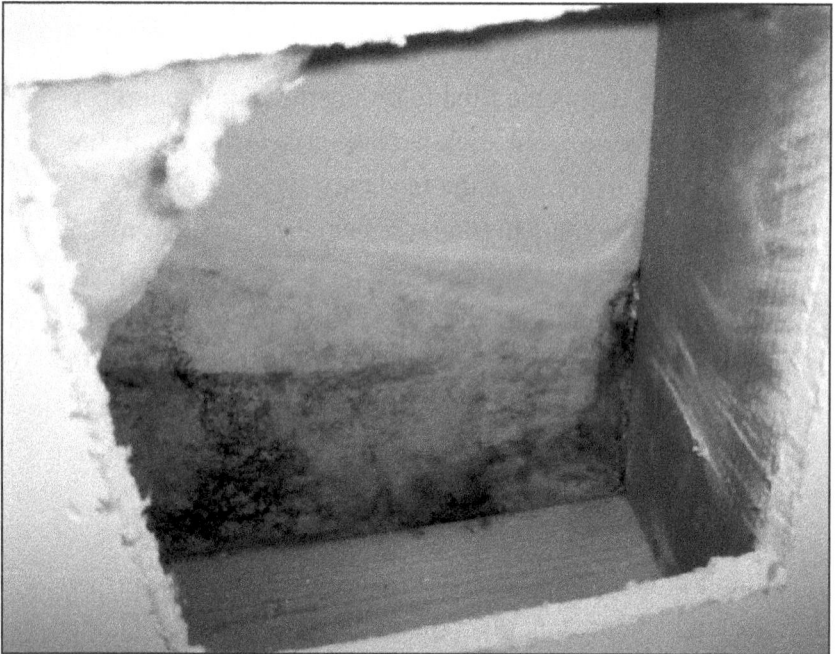

Mold inside a wall cavity.

We Know Nothing

This was a bank owned property. There was a leak while the house was vacant and every room got flooded. The bank said there was no mold. Although air testing did not show mold, my client, the buyer, was still concerned.

We arbitrarily tested some walls. The lab results came back showing mold in every wall. My client decided to not purchase the house. The bank had a painting crew repaint all the walls, claiming it was normal routine. They did not disclose the wall tests and sold the house, as is, to someone else.

Beware of bank foreclosures. Banks may use an intermediate agent to be in charge of the sale. They hide behind the agent and claim they know nothing about the property. They say, "As is," which is fine except they don't always tell you everything they know.

How expensive is it to test for mold?

It depends on how easy it is to find mold that may be hiding. It cost more to test to the point you can be certain there is *not* mold than if mold is readily visible.

The average homeowner, unaware of how a mold inspection should go, calls a few companies and goes with the lowest estimate. That may seem like the reasonable thing to do, but how can a mold inspector quote you a price if he doesn't know how many tests might be required to find the mold or make sure there is no mold?

What you are being quoted is the cost of a few air samples. Do you need air samples? If an inspector finds mold during his visual inspection, you don't.

When calling to get an estimate for testing, ask what a mold inspection company charges for their time and for laboratory fees. Describe why you are calling: Do you see mold? Do you smell mold? Why do you think you have mold? Is it routine because you are buying a property?

To be accurate, testing a house for mold often costs more than the lowest bid. On the flip side it might cost less. If a good inspector finds mold during his visual inspection he doesn't need to do any testing and may end up being the cheapest.

www.academy.healthylivingspaces.com

If you are interested in doing your own testing, check out the on-line courses at www.academy.healthylivingspaces.com. In *Where to Look for Mold and What to Do if You Find It*, I walk you through how to do a mold inspection. *How to Test for Hidden Mold* teaches how to use the WallChek. Courses include where to rent equipment and how to interpret laboratory results. Real life case studies are presented to aid in understanding what's normal and what means there's mold. Learn how collect samples for clearance testing (Post Remediation Verification).

Key Points To Remember From Chapter 2

• Don't bother with self-test kits. You will drive yourself crazy wondering which is it - You have mold the test did not detect or the test is showing you have mold you don't.

• To locate a certified mold inspector, enter your zip code at ACAC.org and look for a Certified Microbial Consult-ant (CMC). The ACAC is the only non-profit that verifies field experience and is accredited by the Engineering Standards Board (ESB).

• Mold is microscopic (invisible without a microscope). Don't cut holes to look for mold. There is a better way to test for hidden mold.

Part 2

MOLD REMEDIATION
MADE SIMPLE

Chapter 3

What Does Not Remove Mold & Why Most Homeowners Are Getting Ripped Off

If any of the following are in an estimate, walk away from using the company. Even if they say, "It's just in case." In case what? They can't remove the mold you are paying them thousands of dollars to remove? Rubbish. Move on.

Bleach

The New York City Department of Health was the first public health organization to provide guidance on how to remediate mold, *Guidelines on Assessment and Remediation of Fungi in Indoor Environments*. The EPA guidelines were copied verbatim from New York.

The first edition that New York published said to use bleach. That has been rescinded. Since 2008, the guidelines say, "Do not use bleach...cleaning should be done using soap or a detergent solution using the gentlest cleaning method that effectively removes the mold. Disinfectants are seldom needed because the removal of fungal growth remains the most effective way to prevent exposure."

The EPA has not updated their guidelines since copying from the original New York edition.

Antimicrobials

Did you know that antibiotic resistant molds and bacteria have been with us since the beginning? Scientists have known this since penicillin was discovered. They tried to solve the problem. They never did. Some species and strains of microbes have evolved, will evolve, and become resistant to current antibiotics. How do you know the antimicrobial used to treat the mold in your home will work a few years from now?

There's so much we don't know about products used to kill microorganisms. Scientists don't even know how common antimicrobials in hand soap work. One thing they know for sure - antimicrobials don't kill *everything*.

It is my experience that remediators who use antimicrobials do not clean as well as they should. They spend their time applying antimicrobials and yet mold is still present after they are finished.

Antimicrobials will not prevent mold. You will not get a guarantee from a mold remediation company because they used antimicrobials. They will encourage you to have them applied and enjoy making money applying them. They will not guarantee that the mold was removed and will never grow back. To prevent mold growth you have to identify and fix the source of moisture. Save money - skip the anti-microbial step and fix the source of the moisture.

Antimicrobials are used because remediators are afraid if they don't use them they will fail the post testing. They don't understand that antimicrobials are not helping them remove mold. It's a crazy cycle – if they fail a job (test results detect mold they missed) they use more the next time.

I'm not trying to be a slave driver. Stop and think about it - you are paying a company to remove mold. Why pay a lot and allow them to try and shortcut the process?

There's one more reason to avoid using antimicrobials. Nothing kills *everything*. The organisms that survive have an advantage. I have clients who had mold in their homes; mold they claim never bothered them until they tried to kill it. They became sick only after they treated the mold. Some still struggle with health issues and hypersensitivity to mold.

I received this email from a reader in Forest, Virginia:

"I reviewed your study of the different mold products (Appendix 2). I used two products for fogging. The yeast growth afterwards in your study caught my attention. I believe each time after I have fogged, especially with mold killer, I created an explosion of yeast that affected me as bad as the mold." (Author's comment: Yeast is a type of fungi, mold.)

Ozone

Ozone is touted to remove everything from mold to pet allergens. It's rubbish. Ozone does not remove mold.

Most people do not understand how ozone works. It burns. It has the same chemical equation for combustion as anything that burns: gasoline, firewood. You have incomplete combustion and residual compounds you didn't have before.

Ozone reacts with things in your home that may cause new odors. In particular, paint, rubber, some types of rugs, carpet backings and synthetic leather are affected by ozone.

Hydrogen Peroxide

An experiment I did in partnership with Los Alamos National Laboratories (See Appendix or my website, www.healthyliving-spaces.com for a copy) has data that shows hydrogen peroxide does not kill mold. In our experiments we used an actual home that had real mold growth. Hydrogen peroxide didn't do much to the mold at all. All that fizzing is fooling you.

Essential Oils

Some natural health professionals swear by a concoction of essential oils. Some have anti-microbial properties. They are a natural defense for the plants they are extracted from, built in pesticides so insects and mold don't eat them.

If you have mold growing in your house, it's too late for prevention. We want to remove the mold, not treat or kill it. The same logic applies to essential oils as conventional antimicrobials – they do not remove mold and are unnecessary.

Essential Gibsons

For example, Kirk had mold in his house. Someone said they could fix his house by killing the mold with essential oils. Afterwards he couldn't enter his house and had to move. He has to keep his Gibson guitars that were in the house sealed in plastic bags. The odor makes him sick.

Some think essential oils are better than conventional antimicrobials because of the notion that natural means non-toxic. Oil is oil, meaning it is a hydrocarbon and hydrocarbons are toxic.

If you must, save them for after the mold is removed. If the place smells like tea tree oil the mold inspector can't do his job and *smell* if the mold is gone.

Air scrubbers (a.k.a. Negative Air Machines)

I wish I had a dollar for every mold remediator that thought bringing in an air scrubber would solve the mold problem.

Air scrubbers do not remove mold! They clean air. So many remediators encourage people to pay for an air scrubber to run a few extra days when a few hours after they finish demolition is sufficient.

Something many mold remediators don't know: One of

the primary reasons for using an air scrubber is to protect workers. Respirators are 99% effective at best. During remediation there may be trillions of spores in the air depending on how carefully the mold is removed. Let's do the math. If one million spores of mold per liter of air are present (a low estimate) and a respirator is 99.9% effective (a high estimate that is rare) a worker is still breathing 10,000 spores per liter of air.

After remediation, the scrubber should be shut off before testing. Don't let the mold inspector test the air while the scrubber is running or you will be testing clean air. Test the air under normal conditions after the contractor turns it off for at least twenty-four hours.

Some remediators will want to run the air scrubber until the laboratory results are back which can be several days after the mold is removed. This results in you paying $100 or more per day per scrubber plus filter changes. Have them shut it off after they are finished.

UV (Ultraviolet Light)

The pigments in mold have light-absorbing molecules that protect the mold from ultraviolet light. Anyone that says UV light kills mold had to have exposed spores to a very strong dosage for a long time. You can't do that to mold in your house because you can't bring the mold out into the open where you can shine a (strong) light on it. Even if you could kill the mold (same old story here) dead mold is still allergenic and potentially toxigenic.

Mold Killers

Read the labels. They can be misleading. They might even say, "Removes mold." If you read more carefully, you will find they either do not remove mold or do not kill every type of mold.

One label I read says it works only when applied to hard, nonporous surfaces. It says to spray the area to be treated and wipe it clean. Hello. You are wiping mold off a hard surface. Yes, that removes mold. You didn't need to treat it because it would have wiped off with soap and water. Hard surfaces are easy to clean. Porous surfaces (wall board) are a different story. Mold growing into walls cannot be wiped off. The walls needs to be cut out.

Read the Material Safety Data Sheets (MSDS). Some products are quite hazardous. It might be worth it if they removed mold but they don't.

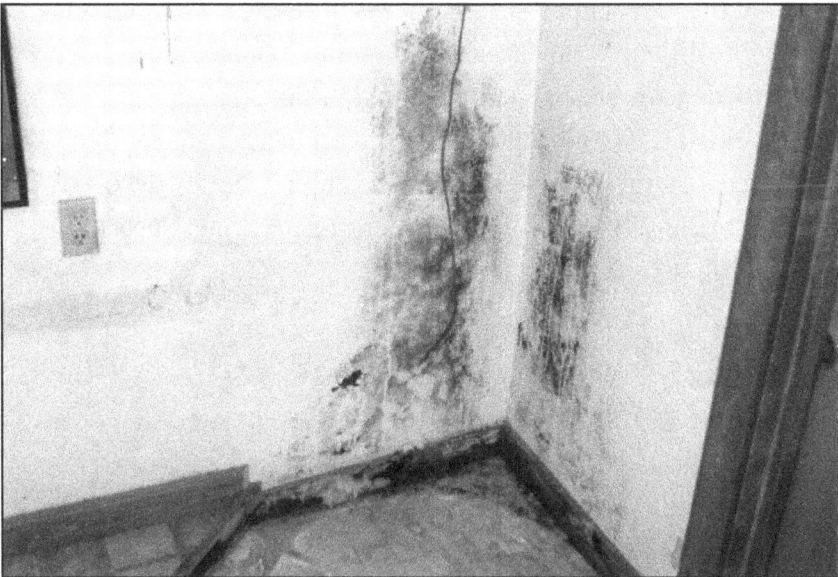

Mold hiding behind cabinets sprayed with a mold killer.

Mold can grow through paint

If you read labels, paints and primers say surfaces must be clean and free of mold and mildew before applying them. Paints are designed to inhibit mold, not encapsulate or cover mold.

I have seen mold grow through paint.

I have seen paint cover mold quite well. More than once I couldn't do a mold inspection because the owners selling a property had painted over mold and claimed it was gone. I had to tell them to sand the paint off since I don't have x-ray vision.

Some selling their homes think they are being clever by painting over mold and not disclosing it. They get caught when painting misses spots that are hard to reach. The mold test detects there is mold and it becomes obvious that paint was used to cover things up. The question arises - what else did they cover up? The paint needs to be sanded off and it is more difficult and expensive to remove the mold.

There are special paint coatings designed to encapsulate mold. If used, they should not contain EPA registered ingredients as these may expose the occupants to low levels of pesticides. Read the MSDS (Material Safety Data Sheet).

Borax

Borax is a mold inhibitor and can be used to treat lumber to prevent termites. (Almost all newer homes are built with framing sill plates treated with arsenic to prevent termites. This also prevents mold.) For untreated wood, once mold has grown, it's too late. The focus should be on removing mold.

Does borax remove mold? It might help with scrubbing but you're making things wet. Mold likes water. It's more effective to scrub things that are dry - spores come off allowing the HEPA air scrubber and HEPA vacuum cleaning you are paying for to capture them.

Some might argue the roots of the mold are embedded into the wood and the wood needs to be treated. Unless wood is rotten, the mycelium (mold roots) is growing only a hair's depth into the surface. Wire brushing is sufficient. There's no need to use borax or treat the wood.

Labels can't tell you what they don't know

Some products sold to kill or remove mold or to remove mold stains, seal the mold with an invisible coating. The consumer and mold remediator has no idea that this is happening.

In partnership with Los Alamos National Laboratories, Healthy Living Spaces discovered this while testing products to see how well they killed or removed mold. Under the microscope we observed the invisible coating that was sealing the mold.

If you want sealed mold, products like this are for you. If you want to make sure mold is removed, these products are not advisable.

If products like this are used, testing may be more difficult (expensive) since the mold is covered up. In my inspections if it's discovered anything other than plain soap and water were used, I suggest having the coating removed similar to if paint were used.

Some coatings off-gas chemicals. I had a project for which

a mold remediator wanted to use a product that we were unsure would affect the air quality in the house. This was a product with a color brochure, a picture of a family on the cover and the words, "non-toxic" and "safe." The remediator wanted to use it because it claimed it could remove mold by fogging.

We contacted the manufacturer and proposed that we would test the air in the home before and after the house was treated. We proposed that if chemicals from the treatment showed up in the air, they would be responsible for restoring the home to pre-treatment conditions. The manufacturer declined to participate.

One manufacturer I contacted didn't know what kind of respiratory protection should be worn. They said, "Respirator," then added, "Probably a VOC (vapor chemical) respirator." An acid vapor was produced for which neither type of respirator provides protection.

Some products leave behind ammonium quaternary salts. The manufacturer may say it's a small amount; ammonium quaternary is toxic, even in small amounts.

New problems

I thought the idea of getting rid of mold was to have a clean, safe, healthy living environment. Who wants new problems? Who wants to pay to have them? Take chemical odors from antimicrobials. How long does it take for these odors to go away? In one real estate transaction, not fast enough for the buyers.

The seller chose a remediation company that likes to use

antimicrobials. This particular antimicrobial has a base of isopropyl alcohol. I told the remediation company not to use it and they said they wouldn't. The workers forgot and used it anyway. The deal was killed because the buyer didn't like the residual odor. It didn't help that workers thought that if a little helps, then using a lot must help even more.

In another example, the mold remediator used a "natural" antimicrobial, one that contains an essential oil. The smell of the essential oil is so strong the manufacturer adds an artificial fragrance, limonene, to lessen the odor of the essential oil.

After the mold remediation company used it, the homeowner could not tolerate the new odor. It took months of airing out the house before they got used to it. In the meantime the remediator washed down all the walls and cleaned the HVAC system several times in an effort to remove as much of the odor as possible.

There are always people dreaming up the next thing to try and kill or treat mold. It's time consuming to keep up with it all. In the end you get the idea - there is one way to remove mold - physical labor. That's why mold remediation is expensive. Disinfecting, ozonating, antimicrobials and killing mold, do not remove mold.

A lot of remediation companies think they can short cut the process but charge you rates as if they had worked hard. Now you know better.

Bleach Please

Here's a recommendation from a mold *inspection* company that recommends bleach:

"Sanitize the cleaned structure with a 7% hydrogen

peroxide or a 5:1 solution of bleach. Allow a minimum contact time of 20 minutes, during which time the structure members are to be kept visibly wet with the sanitizing agent".

Why would we need to sanitize a clean structure? If the mold was removed and the structure is clean there should be no mold to sanitize. They are making things wet and they want you to do it twice. As one client of mine said, "No point in adding more liquid. Dry it out and remove the mold."

If this is in the mold remediation company's estimate I would suggest they go back to the mold inspector and ask the mold inspector to revise his recommendations.

Key Point To Remember From Chapter 3

- Everyone is trying to dream up the next big thing to kill mold. None of these remove mold. Next, we'll cover the details on how mold can and should be removed.

Chapter 4

WHAT WORKS

Remember what are we trying to accomplish. (Hint: It's not to kill the mold.)

Screwdriver

You may need a screwdriver, pliers, wrench or similar tools. If, for example, mold is in a kitchen or bathroom, some cabinets or vanities may need to be removed. They are often in the way of cutting out mold on walls behind them. Sometimes it's a toilet, bathtub, dishwasher or hot water heater that needs to be removed. Often cabinets have mold on the back or bottom sides in places not visible until they are removed.

Razor blade, fitted saw, pry-bar

The idea is to minimize the amount of dust and mold disturbed because it's much easier to clean up a mess if it can be minimized. The razor blade knife is used to carefully cut out wallboard instead of using a hammer. Fitted saws have vacuum attachments that collect dust as they cut. The pry-bar is for carefully pulling drywall off walls after the wall has been scored with the razor or saw.

Trash Bags

As soon as pieces of moldy drywall, insulation or wood are removed, the debris should be placed in large, contractor grade trash bags.

Wire-brush

After drywall is removed the wood should be wire-brushed or sanded. The brush works better than sanding in areas that have corners such as the bottom of sill plates and the edges of wood framing. No special mold remediation brush is required. Use a wire brush found in the paint department at the hardware store.

HEPA Vacuum

Clean as you go. The vacuum should be held near the wire-brush when brushing. The definition of HEPA is High-efficiency Particulate Arrestance. It means that 99.97% of what

goes into the vacuum stays in the vacuum instead of blowing out the bag.

Dish soap, pail and rags

This is what the, *Guidelines on Assessment and Remediation of
Fungi in Indoor Environments,* means where it says, "Use the
gentlest detergent possible." It worked for cleaning oil off birds in
oil spills and it works for cleaning mold. I prefer non-fragrant soap
so we can smell if the mold is gone.

HEPA Air Scrubber

It's as much work to remove mold, as it is to prepare a house
for mold remediation. You want to prevent dust from escap-
ing into other places of the house. It's called containment and
it is why mold remediation can be expensive.

Containment requires an air scrubber (also called a negative air machine). The air scrubber is not used to scrub air.
The fan inside it is used to exhaust air from the work area
to outside of the house. This creates suction in the work
area. To be effective, the scrubber must be connected to an
exhaust duct that goes outdoors through a window or door
opening. The scrubber should be turned on *before* starting
work. Don't pick up a screwdriver to remove cabinets until
the scrubber is running.

In the old days, contractors placed a box fan in the window fac-
ing outward and made a tight fit between the fan and window

frame using duct tape and plastic. This may work for do-it-your-selfers with small work areas.

In detail, the steps are:

Set up "Containment"

Unless the mold is isolated to one room and the door can be closed, you will have to hang plastic from the floor to ceiling to create a work area. The air scrubber should be placed in the middle of the work area and the exhaust duct from the scrubber should go outside though a door or window.

Issue to watch for: Some contractors do not exhaust the scrubber outside. Some exhaust it to another room in the house or run it without an exhaust duct attached.

Issue to watch for: Some contractors bring the scrubber in at the end of the job thinking it's to clean the air. It is not to clean the air – it's to create a negative air pressure in the work area. Bringing it in afterwards is a waste of money.

Pull out what's in the way

Chances are, most of the mold is hidden inside walls or ceiling cavities. If for example, the leak happened in the kitchen or bathroom there may be cabinets in the way that need to be pulled.

Cut out moldy walls and ceilings

Mold is microscopic. Cut drywall out two feet past from where it looks moldy or wet or stained on the backside. Going two feet past visible mold or staining is a safe bet.

Issue to watch for: Some contractors will cut out walls to the exact spot mold is visible and stop. They don't go an inch past it. Others cut out too much. You might be paying by the square foot. If this is the case do not let them cut out too much or cut too little.

Anything rotten should be removed. This may mean cutting out sections of flooring, sill plates (the bottom framing on walls), plywood on exterior walls, roof decking. Some contractors might tell you it's easier for them to cut something out than clean it. That's great, the more cut out the better.

Issue to watch for: Some contractors don't cut rot out. They may try a variety of things such as sanding, cleaning or sealing rotten wood or spraying it with something. Often you can tell just by looking that something's not right.

Sand and wire-brush

The remaining wood (and hard surfaces such as block and concrete) should be sanded and wire-brushed. A wire brush gets into nooks and crannies better than sanding. If it's too difficult to brush, it might be necessary to remove the material instead of clean it.

Clean

HEPA vacuum everything: ceiling, walls, framing, floor, inside wall cavities. A shop-vac can be used if the vacuum is outside with the hose feed through the window.

After vacuuming, damp wipe everything using plain soap and water. All of the mold should have been removed. Bleach is poor for cleaning because it does not have a surfactant. The ions in bleach repel from a surface, like trying to touch two magnets together. Lots of rags are required. Dirty rags should not go back into the cleaning solution.

Things should look and smell clean or you've missed something. That's what testing and post inspections by the mold inspector are for.

That's the process. If anyone tries to convince you there is a better way, take a moment, consider it, then let it go and remember the basics: Mold is either removed or not. If people would stop getting caught up in hi-tech products and gizmos to *treat* mold, they would realize these do not remove mold and how simple the science of removing mold really is.

Cleaning your stuff

Questions often asked include, "Should I clean the contents? How do I clean my stuff?" It's difficult to say how critical it is to clean the contents. Often it's not everything that is cleaned, only items that were in close proximity to the mold. It depends on how moldy the house was, where the mold

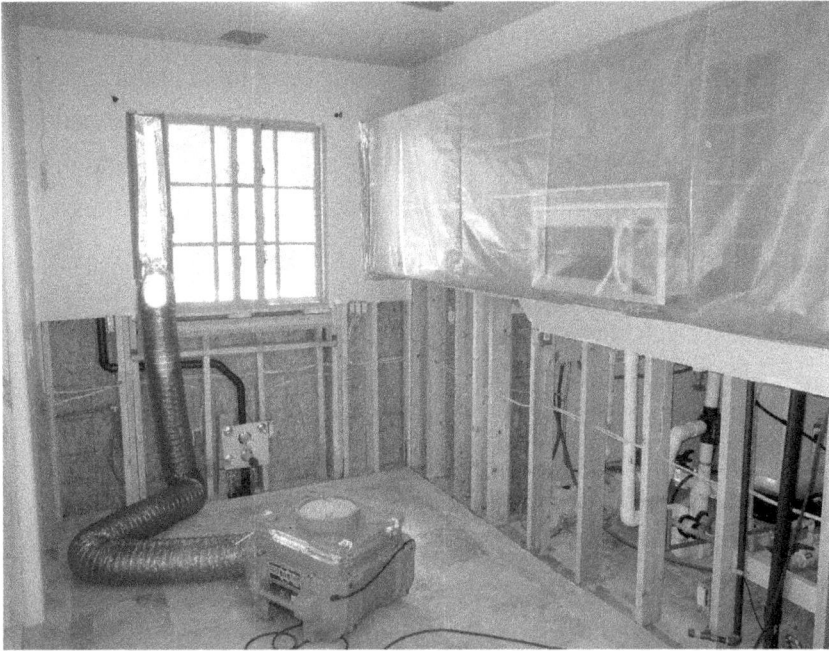

A good job. Notice the plastic covering the cabinets, the air scrubber is exhausted out the window, sections of walls have been removed, and the room is clean.

was, and how sensitive people are.

To begin, separate what got wet and has visible mold growing on it vs. items that were simply in the same room with mold. If you can see mold or something smells like mold - throw it away.

If something did not get wet, mold cannot grow on it. What you are cleaning are spores and fragments that settled out in the dust. They cannot grow unless they get wet. Clean your things the way you normally clean something that is dusty - soap and water, laundry with regular laundry soap, vacuum, mop. Take the couch and bedding outdoors and beat them with a stick (wearing a respirator). Do not use bleach, chemicals or biocides. They are not going to help clean.

You can't see what you are cleaning so have patience. Sensitive people are bothered by a little bit of mold in the dust; others don't seem to be bothered at all. Somewhere in between is common sense. The following is a stripped down version of a cleaning protocol. Call or email Healthy Living Spaces for the details.

Get the Spring-cleaning tools: bucket of soap and water; vacuum cleaner, and if possible, a compressed air hose or leaf blower. Organize by the type of material:
• Porous stuff (books, cloths, bedding)
• Semi-porous (wood furniture)
• Non-porous (glass, metal)

Take things outside to clean them. Pack cleaned items in boxes and wait to bring them back into the house until after the house is cleaned. Clean the house the same way - vacuuming and damp-wiping.

Anything that can be washed should be washed. Washing is more effective than vacuuming and wiping.

Hard items are easy to clean - plastic, metal, wood, glass - wipe down with soap and water or wash.

Cloths are easy. Use regular laundry soap.

The compressed air hose (or leaf blower) should be used with caution - it can break things if you blow too hard. It helps clean the nooks and crannies on stuff were a vacuum or damp wipe can't reach. Your TV or stereo are examples.

The sequence is as follows. If you submerge an item and wash it you may skip all this:
• Blow with compressed air hose or leaf blower
• Vacuum with HEPA vacuum (or vacuum outside)
• Damp-wipe with soap and water.

It's a big job so get family members and friends to help. People short cut the process doing the best they can. Sometimes you can't clean things outside. This is just an outline.

Professional remediators may give you an estimate to clean the contents. They *never* do it the way it's supposed to be done and charge a fortune. Don't waste your money.

Part 3

How to Save Money

Chapter 5

1ˢᵀ Round draft - Weed Out the Bad Guys

The first thing that will save you money is to avoid using a company that treats mold instead of removes it. Don't waste your money. If any of the following are in an estimate, do not use that company. Don't just ask the company to remove them from the estimate and not to use them. You are asking for trouble. The following are red flags. Chances are they are not use to cleaning as well because they are use to relying on the myth that these help remove mold when they don't. Walk away from a company that uses or has any of the following words in their estimate:

Antimicrobial
Disinfectant
EPA registered
Bleach

Sanitize
Ozone
Fogging
Sealants
Stain remover

Here's an example on how you can save $5,000 by not using a company. The estimate reads:

"Kill The Mold: Disinfection and sterilization of entire attic via fogging/ atomization with a disinfectant to kill airborne spores prior to removal of contaminated materials."

Line items in the estimate included:

Prep the house
Kill the mold
Remove the stains with a stain remover
Kill the roots to prevent reoccurrence
Ozonation to oxidize any remaining hidden spores
Apply inhibitory salt
Clean up our mess

Why would you need to kill mold prior to removing it? Why would you need to ozonate hidden spores after killing the rest of the mold? This seems to admit that the disinfection, sterilization and fogging steps did not work. Why would you need to apply salts to prevent future mold if the sterilization process worked? Nothing in the estimate talks about removing the mold (sanding, wire brushing and so forth).

If we subtract the killing and sanitizing steps, you can almost subtract the entire estimate. The only items left are "Prepping the House" and "Cleaning Up Our Mess".

Estimates like the one above are not isolated to certain cities and states. Here's an estimate from a different company on the opposite side of the country. This remediation company took an air sample, found elevated levels of mold and proposed the following. Yes, the remediation company also did the testing:

"A MOLD ERADICATION, ODOR CLEANSING & SANITIZATION PROCESS. INCLUDES:

1 FOGGING

2 SURFACE APPLICATION TO VISIBLE MOLD USING EXCLUSIVE SOLUTION TO ERADICATE MOLD ROOTS AND MOLD STAINS ON HARD SURFACES

3 INSTALL EXCLUSIVE SANITIZER / ODOR MACHINE / HEPA VACCUM"

There is no mention of scrubbing, sanding, wire brushing or anything related to *removing* mold. The total cost is $3,500. I called the remediator and asked, "If my client lets you do it your way and the air samples still show elevated levels of mold, are you going to be responsible and remove the mold the proper way?"

"No," they said, "Mold is everywhere." After a page of Limitations & Exclusions, the end of the estimate stated, "No warranty is made."

Guarantees to Beware

Beware of: *"We guarantee to beat any other contractors price if it is itemized and duplicated exactly."* You don't want do duplicate a bad estimate! Will the estimate remove the mold? If so, take it. If it's because the mold is being treated (cost less than removing), don't.

Beware of: *"We guarantee that mold will not grow on any areas treated."* This means they are treating mold instead of removing it.

Beware of: *"Once we are finished, the home that was treated will pass a mold test."* The key word is treated. Also, if they seem that confident about passing a mold test afterwards, you might ask more questions about what they will be doing. Even the best mold remediation companies have, on occasion, failed the test afterwards.

Key Points To Remember From Chapter 5

• The only chemicals used should be plain soap and water. A simple thing to do is to ask the remediator if any of the products he intends to use has an EPA registration. Nothing should be used that has to be registered with the EPA.

• Beware of estimates with, "Antimicrobial." It won't remove mold and is a red flag.

• Beware of guarantees. The remediation company may start using language like, "Mold is everywhere," or "We can't give you a sterile house," after charging you thousands of dollars.

Chapter 6

ROUND 2 – WHOM CAN YOU TRUST?

In the end you're going to have to trust who does the work, just like you trust the roofer. It's a choice a customer makes. If a customer wants to pass a mold test because they are selling their house and have a remediator promising that no matter what, they will pass the mold test afterwards, they may choose different than someone buying a house or living in a house who want to make sure the mold is removed instead of being covered up or treated.

Be cautious about estimates with a single price for everything

When you see a mold remediation estimate that is only one page and at the bottom it says exactly $20,000 and zero cents, consider, how did they estimate that? Often they pull it out of a hat. In the end they may charge you the same or more. After starting the job they may say, "We are going to exceed our estimate." You might tell them to stop. Besides money down the drain, a good remediation company is not going to want to take over the mess.

Be cautious about, "We'll do it for ½ the price."

One company tells customers, "Give me the cheapest estimate and I'll do it for half." Alarm bells should go off. How can they do this? Why would you hire them? It doesn't sound right. People do.

Preferred Service Providers (PSP)

Now things get tricky. Franchised water damage and mold remediation companies have agreements with insurance companies. The headquarters of the franchises went to insurance companies and said, "If you give us all your work, we will work for lower prices than the established price list." All of a sudden you have an issue where the customer thinks they are getting a good job but the remediation company must be cutting corners. The remediation company cannot work for those prices. The insurance company might tell you the quality of the work is the same. How would you know? It's like buying a piece of meat at the market - It says, "Organic, grass-fed." You don't really know that it's fed organic grass.

It's not always the cheapest company working under such agreements. Sometimes it is the most expensive. You can't tell by the cost of the estimate or the name of the company.

Ask your insurance. They are called Preferred Service Providers (PSP). PSPs have special pricing arrangements with insurance companies. It's a conflict of interest. If your insurance wants to refer you to a good company, that's great. Your insurance company should give you a list, a complete list, not a list of companies that give them discounts.

Your insurance company cannot make you use a company. If you read your policy, you may pick whom ever you choose.

Beware of this Guarantee:

When you call your insurance 800 number, your insurance may say, "If you work with one of our preferred service providers we will give you a five year warranty."

What they mean is they will warranty the repairs. They will not warranty that the mold was removed. If I go back later, test for mold and find it, the insurance company will not pay to have the mold removed.

"We have offices in three states"

Having a lot of offices does not make a company better. For example, there was a house where a pipe leaked in the kitchen and water flowed into the living room. The remediation company, who had offices in three states, removed a few of the cabinets in the kitchen and some of the walls in the living room. They called me to do an inspection after they were finished.

I found mold in the living room on the backside of the office wall. The office shares a wall with the living room. They said they did not want to expand the job to include the office. I told them I wish the owner didn't have to have the office remediated either but mold is mold. They were supposed to be removing it all, so unless the owner told them to stop, they should have continued.

I returned for another inspection and smelled something coming from the kitchen. Instead of removing all of the cabinets they removed only the ones they thought got wet. I found mold on some cabinets and told them to take them out.

I returned for a third inspection and noticed mold behind the doorframe to the office. I had told the company to remove the doorframe to the office when they removed part of the office wall. They did not listen. I also found mold in the kitchen on the wall behind where the additional cabinets had been removed.

At this point the mold remediation company was furious with me. "We never have a problem passing a mold inspection," they said. "You are doing something wrong."

I emailed the manager at the corporate office in another state pictures of the mold. At first he was reluctant. He finally agreed, "Yes, it is mold. We will remove it."

I don't understand why I am the bad guy. I drove an hour each way to do the inspection three times. In the end they cleaned it up. I wonder how many homes in three states still have mold after this company was paid to remove it.

The bigger they are...

Bigger does not mean better. This is a story about a government building with people complaining about mold odors and being sick for years. Bids were taken to remove the mold. The largest company won the bid.

The mold was in a wall between a bathroom and the offices. A pipe leaked inside a wall behind a toilet. The remediation company was supposed to remove both sides of the walls (office and bathroom). They called me to do an inspection when they were finished.

I found they had re-built everything. I could not do an inspection. I tested the wall again. I was suspicious because the tile inside the bathroom looked the same as it probably did fifty years ago. The test results showed there was still mold in the wall.

It turned out they only removed the office side of the walls. They didn't want to remove the bathroom side because they would have had to close the bathroom. When I told them the test results they asked how dangerous the mold was. They asked if they could leave it in the wall instead of removing it. Keep in mind that taxpayers paid tens of thousands of dollars to this company (the cost including some HVAC work was over $100,000) and people had been sick and complaining for years.

As far as I know they did nothing.

Chapter 7

READ THE ESTIMATE

You should have narrowed your choice to a company that is going to remove mold, not treat it and one that is not giving you the lowest estimate to get the job. Let's make sure you get what you pay for. The following are ways of making sure nothing falls in the cracks. It's nice if you can talk to the owner of the company instead of an estimator. They should explain the process and what they plan to do. At the end of the day, pick the company you feel most comfortable with.

Warning: Some of the following involves math. If math seems tedious, ask the remediator to do it. Ask your mold inspector to help you.

Software Games

Many remediation companies use a piece of software developed to work with insurance companies. The software company works with insurance companies to program a price for each line item. There is a price for removing drywall, renting equipment, sanding, cleaning, removing cabinets, and so forth.

The prices change every month and the remediation companies are supposed to adhere to them. They download the price list. It's the same for every insurance company – there is only one price list. The insurance and software companies claim there is a formula for labor hours and construction material prices but it doesn't make sense. The prices go back and forth.

When they come to give an estimate the remediation company will take measurements. These are not measurements of how much mold there is – you can not tell how much mold is hidden until you start the work. These are measurements of the room. The remediation company plugs the square footage of the walls, ceiling and floors of the room into the program. It allows them to go back after they are finished, measure what was actually done and change the estimate.

Some remediators do not keep track of what is done. They may hand you the same estimate at the end of the job as the final bill. You cannot tell from an estimate what was done or where there was mold.

Air Scrubbers
(also know as Negative Air Fans)

Remediation companies charge $100 or more per scrubber, per day. The more days a scrubber runs, the more money they make. On top of that are fees for changing filters, setting up the equipment, taking down and decontaminating equipment. This adds up to be significant. The cost of "containment" can be thousands of dollars and half the cost of the project.

For example, the cost of renting one air scrubber for four days is approximately $1,200. Some projects take longer. A new machine with new filters can be purchased for that.

LINE ITEM DESCRIPTION	QTY	UNIT COST	ACV (Actual Cash Value)
Neg Air fan / Scrubber	4 Days	$100	$400
Add for HEPA filter	1	$220	$220
Add for primary filter changes (3 per day)	12	$30	$360
Add for secondary filter changes (1 per day)	4	$12	$48
Equipment set-up, take down and monitoring0.75 hours for 4 days	3 Hours	$42 / HR	$126
Equipment decontamination per piece of equipment	1	$40	$40
Total cost for renting one air scrubber / neg air machine for 4 days:			**$1,194**

The cost of renting one air scrubber for four days.

I wonder who started the idea of renting air scrubbers. A builder does not charge a homeowner to rent his power tools. A painter does not charge $100 per day to rent their power sprayers. I find it odd that insurance companies often will not pay for mold remediation yet don't seem to care how the money is spent when they do.

Check the number of scrubbers (neg air fans)

Look on the estimate for how many air scrubbers are estimated. At least one scrubber is required in each work area. If you know only one will be used you can skip this section. Sometimes if a remediation company knows insurance is paying, they will specify more than what is necessary, more than one scrubber per work area.

If more than one scrubber is to be used, ask how the number of scrubbers required was calculated. A scrubber has a maximum number of cubic feet of airflow per minute (CFM). Calculate the volume of the work area (length X width X ceiling height). These dimensions are usually in the drawing the remediator made in the estimate. Multiple this volume by four (the number of air changes per hour required) and divide by 60 (minutes per hour). This is the CFM needed from a scrubber. It is either adequate or a second scrubber is required.

For example, a kitchen 20 x 10 feet with 10 foot ceiling has a volume of 2,000 cubic feet. A scrubber with a minimum of 133 CMF is required. Even the smallest scrubber on the market is rated at 600 CFM. One scrubber is enough.

Check the number of days the scrubber will be used.

A typical remediation is three days: one for set up, one for demolition, one for final cleaning. Since the first day will be spent hanging plastic, covering the floor with a protective covering and so forth, the scrubber may not be used on that day.

Ask the remediator if they plan on leaving the scrubber on after they are finished while you wait for test results from the laboratory. You can save money by turning the scrubber off while you wait for lab test results. You lived in your house before without one. Why the sudden need to have an air scrubber running 24/7 if the remediator is confident a good job was done removing the mold?

Consider telling the remediator you don't want a new HEPA filter installed.

There are two reasons for this:

A new filter is $200-$300 per machine installed. You will never know if a new HEPA filter was installed. You're going to have to take their word for it. When finished, companies throw the machines on the truck. To install a new HEPA filter requires time and a screwdriver. If they are busy and need the machine on another job, chances are the filter is not going to be changed.

The machine does not need to have a new HEPA filter. Some remediators may say the HEPA filter needs to be changed to avoid the potential liability of contaminating your house with dust from the last job. If the machine contaminates a house it is not because the HEPA filter is dirty. The issue is either inside the machine is dirty or the filter is not a true HEPA. If you test the scrubber with a laser particle counter you might find the scrubber is not HEPA even with a new

filter installed. Changing the filter won't improve perform-
ance. There will be contamination coming out of the machine
from other jobs unless every component inside the machine
is washed. The solution is to always exhaust the scrubber
outdoors. Never let a remediator exhaust it into another
room of the house.

Check the square footage of the line item, "HEPA Vacuuming – Detailed"

This can be a big-ticket item. It's based on the combined
square footage of the walls and ceilings, not just the floor.
The cost of vacuuming per square foot might seem small
(50 to 60 cents) but multiplied by a thousand square-feet it
becomes $500 to $600.

To put it in perspective, if you have a room that's 300
square feet with eight-foot ceilings, it would cost $517 to
vacuum. That is not the total cost to clean. There is another
line item for wiping the walls, ceiling, and floors with soap
and water (or an antimicrobial). If the work area extends to
other areas of the house, the cost is increased.

A HEPA vacuum is still just a vacuum. We want to make
the area as small as possible. Besides being cheaper to clean,
its easier to clean smaller areas. *Don't let the remediator
treat the entire room as one big work area.* If mold is
growing on only one side of the room, have them isolate
that part of the room by hanging plastic floor to ceiling
across the middle of the room. Have them update the drawing in the estimate to reflect the new dimensions.

Check the size (square footage) of the line item, "Containment Barrier / Airlock / Decon Chamber"

Decon chambers are pass-through booths that you walk through to go between the work area and the rest of the house. Some estimates have a line item for cleaning the decon chamber. It's based on the square footage of the "Containment Barrier / Airlock / Decon-Chamber". Similar to the line item, "HEPA Vacuuming – Detailed", they will charge you to vacuum and clean it when there are done. Check that the decon chamber is of a reasonable size. They only need to be a few square feet.

The decon chamber gets thrown away anyhow. You paid for it in another line item.

Check how many square feet of material are to be removed

Note how many square feet of drywall and other materials are to be cut out and removed. The removal of drywall and insulation are not big-ticket items. The issue is cutting out too much or too little to start with.

One homeowner had half his garage ceiling removed even though there was only mold over the top of the garage door. The remediator did not read the mold inspection report. The remediator was only supposed to remove the wall above the top of the garage door. The client had to rebuild half his garage ceiling and the remediation company charged him mold remediation rates, even though the garage ceiling did not have mold.

Really?

This was a small job, a coat closet. The company used two of the biggest air scrubbers money can buy. They probably used more scrubbers than necessary because insurance was paying.

When I came to do the final testing, I found the scrubbers were still running. I explained that if I was going to test the air, the scrubbers had to be off. Otherwise I am testing filtered air.

The air scrubbers were exhausting into the family room. I tested the scrubbers with a laser particle counter. They were removing only 60% of the particles passing through them instead of 99%, which is the HEPA standard. The scrubbers were contaminating the home with dust and mold from previous jobs.

I returned a few days later and found the scrubbers still running, still exhausting into the family room. Meanwhile, they charged the client an additional $1,250 ($125 per scrubber, per day, for five additional days).

I could smell bleach. Although the supervisor said they would not use bleach, the worker decided to use a little, "Just in case."

This was a Preferred Service Provider company.

It's More than Drywall

Reading through the narrative of one estimate, I noticed what I thought was an error: The remediation company proposed to use the HEPA air scrubber *after* removing the moldy drywall.

"Why aren't you using the air scrubber *during* demolition?" I asked.

"Because drywall is not a regulated hazardous material," they said.

"Mold is not a regulated hazardous material," I said. "Why use the scrubber at all?"

"Because the home owner wants us to," they said. "But we don't need to use one while the drywall is being removed."

I explained that the purpose of an air scrubber is to create a negative air pressure and keep dust from getting into the rest of the house, not to clean the air after work is done. Bringing the scrubber in at the end of the job is a waste of money. This raised red flags. I told my client to find someone else to do the work.

Watch for excessive line items

To be fair, the software used when working with insurance companies has a set price list. The remediator enters the square footage. They can't adjust the price too much. If you spot these items ahead of time perhaps you can find a cheaper way to have them done.

An example is carpet. The carpet, which was in a room with mold on the walls, was not moldy. To remove 170 square feet of carpet, at a unit price of 37 cents per square foot, cost $63. To dispose of the carpet was another line item, $150. The trash bill was another line item.

How many hours does it take to remove a small area of carpet? If we estimate thirty minutes that's $126 per hour plus the disposal fee of $150. They aren't treating the carpet. They roll it up, carry it out, and throw it into the dumpster.

The homeowner could have rolled up the carpet and saved $200. The homeowner would not have been in any danger of being exposed to mold. They could have thrown the carpet into the dumpster the remediator was bringing. The dumpster was another line item.

Should you have the ducts cleaned?

Maybe. It may be worth it if they have never been cleaned.

Duct cleaning only works for metal ducts. Ducts made out of fiberboard should be removed if contaminated with mold growth. Flex ducts are too difficult to effectively clean.

If the furnace sits on a platform and there is a cavity under the furnace being used as a return air plenum, it's often filthy under there. There can be a big difference cleaning it. Some duct cleaning companies miss it. You could vacuum it yourself.

Do not use sanitizers. They do not remove mold, are a waste of money and can be toxic.

If the liner inside the furnace or air-conditioning blower compartment is burnt or covered in dust it should be replaced. Use foil and foil tape.

Duct cleaning estimates are based on the number of ducts cleaned. The principle is that time is spent on each duct. You need to supervise. Often workers are in a hurry. Duct cleaning is only effective if time is spent putting elbow grease into each one.

Is there a guarantee?

What happens if the work does not pass the mold test afterwards? Who pays for the mold inspector to come back twice? A good mold remediator will guarantee passing the mold test. They will pay if the mold inspector has to come back and re-test because they missed spots.

There are times it's not the mold remediator's fault. Sometimes mold is hidden in a way they can't be blamed for missing it. Ask your mold inspector how they will determine when it's the remediator's fault for missing mold and when there's no way the remediator could have known there was additional mold hiding.

Chapter 8

SUPERVISE THE WORKERS

This section is about more than saving money – it's about making sure you get what you pay for and the job is done right. Although you should have weeded out the bad guys, sometimes, something goes wrong. It's a good idea to supervise the job. At least be present at the beginning until you are confident the company is doing what they said they would, the way they said they would. Mold remediation is not magic. You might be surprised at how straightforward and common sense it can be.

Don't let workers scare or intimidate you. Sometimes they post warning signs at the entry to the work area saying keep out. Remind them it is your property and that you had mold before they got there. Stay out during activities that generate dust. Go in after the dust settles. The end of the day is a good time. Wear a respirator. You may want a camera, tape measure and notebook.

Sneaky Business

I showed up to do the post inspection at the same time the remediator was wheeling in the air scrubber. I was a bit confused and asked what they were doing.

"Setting up the air scrubber," they said.

I wondered to myself, are they just setting it in now? Was it not used during demolition? Things look clean. I'm ready to test.

They got defensive and insisted that was how things are supposed to be done. (Bring the scrubber in at the end of the job to clean the air). I told them to take it away and not charge my client for it.

Day 1: What to look for

Log Book

This is a good time to check to see if there is a logbook. It should be used to keep track of items that are disposed of: filters that are changed, respirator changes, PPE (Personal Protective Equipment) disposable suits and so forth. It should keep a record of line items that you are charged for by the hour such as time spent monitoring equipment, changing filters and decontaminating equipment. If the remediation company gripes about keeping track of things, ask how they are going to calculate a final bill. Ask if they are going to hand you the original estimate verbatim.

I've come to the conclusion that having mold remediation done is like going to the dealership to get your car repaired – there are line items on your bill that are automatically added, shop fees, disposal fees, a fixed number of hours on the estimate to make repairs even although the technician may have taken less hours to do the work. In the end you may just have to trust the remediator. It might be hard to find one willing to work under this kind of supervision.

Here's an example of a logbook. There should be a new page each day.

LOG BOOK for: _____ **(Address)**   **DATE:**
CONSUMABLES / HOURS WORKED

LINE ITEM	HOURS	QTY	COMMENTS
Content Manipulation			
Equipment Set-up / Take –down			
Supervisor			
PPE (Disposable Suit Discarded)			
Respirator cartridge changed HEPA only type filter			
Respirator cartridge changed HEPA/Vapor Gas type filter			

Sample logbook to keep track of used supplies and hours worked

Containment

The first thing a remediator should do is set up the containment. This includes the air scrubber (negative air machine). You are likely paying $1,000 or more to have containment. Set things up correctly and it doesn't matter if a

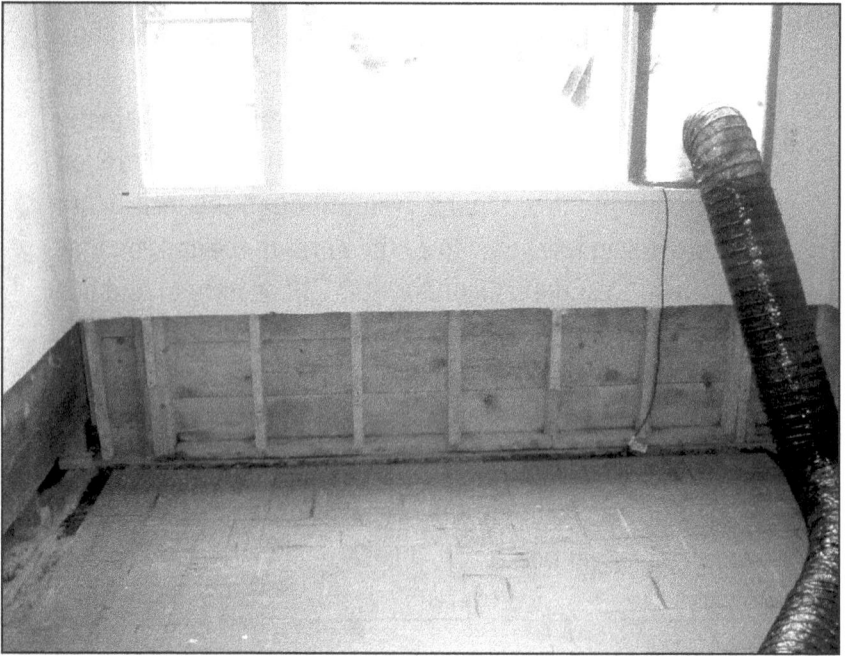

Air scrubber duct going out a window in order to create a negative air pressure (suction) in the work area.

bomb explodes, all the dust is contained; set things up wrong, it's a waste of money.

Check how big the containment is. Does it need to be the entire room? The software program generated an estimate based on the square feet of walls, ceiling and floor that need to be cleaned. The smaller the containment, the smaller the area there is to clean. If they can move the contents to one side of the room and hang plastic floor to ceiling across the middle of it, the cost of HEPA vacuuming and damp-wiping at the end of the job is cut in half.

The scrubber needs to be exhausted outside via a duct through a door or window.

After the scrubber is turned on the remediator should verify there is an adequate negative air pressure created. This is done with a pressure gauge. I use a digital Pressure and Flow meter made by the Energy Conservatory. There should be a minimum negative pressure of 0.02 inches of water column (5 Pascal) in the work area relative to outside the work area (the rest or the house). Readings should be entered into the logbook with a separate page for each scrubber (negative air fan) each day.

LOG BOOK for: _____ (Address)   **DATE:**

NEG AIR FAN / SCRUBBER LOG SHEET

Containment Area: (Kitchen / Bathroom / Family Room / Bedroom / Other)

Negative air fan / scrubber #   (If more than one scrubber)

Air scrubber running today?   (Y/N)

Pressure difference between work area containment and outside containment
_____(Inches of water or Pascal)

Primary filters changed	QTY:
Secondary filters changed	QTY:
Technician Hours	HOURS:
Supervisor Hours	HOURS:
COMMENTS:	

Sample logbook for air scrubber and monitoring pressure inside containment

Check the equipment

How do you know the HEPA air scrubber you are paying for is HEPA? Ask them to check it using a laser particle counter. They should measure the level of particles in the room air and

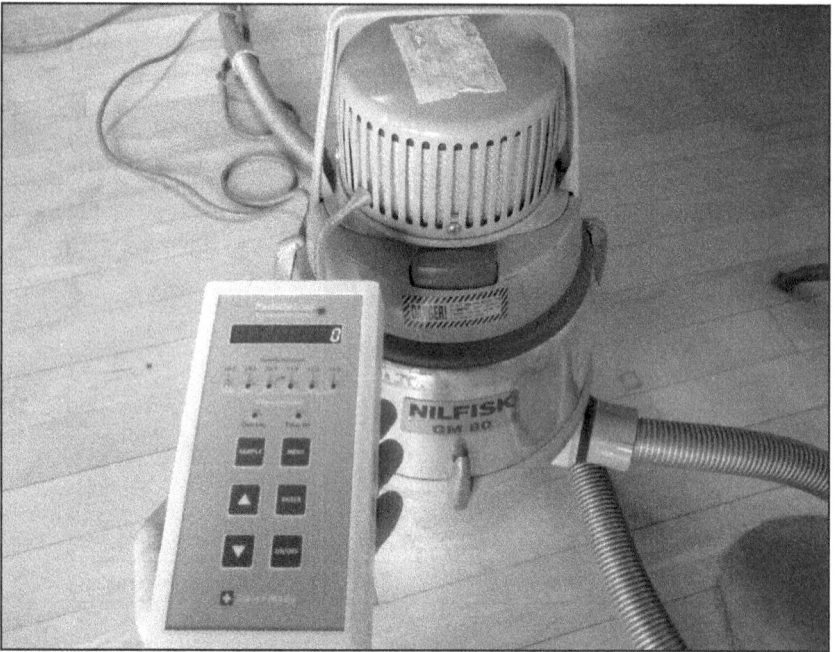

Checking a HEPA vacuum cleaner with a laser particle counter. Note the zero particle reading at the exhaust of the vacuum.

then hold the particle counter near the exhaust of the air scrubber. The definition of HEPA is a 99.97 % reduction in particles. You may need a consultant (mold inspector) to perform the test. The remediator may not own a laser particle counter or be familiar with the procedure. (The standard, *Portable High Efficiency Air Filtration Device Field Testing and Validation Standard,* under development by the Indoor Environmental Standard Organization, will be helpful when it's completed.)

If the scrubber is not operating at 99% try using foil tape to seal the edges of the machine around the pre-filters. If it still does not perform to HEPA standards, consider allowing them to use it. Make sure it's exhausted out a window and ask them to not bill you for a HEPA air scrubber.

The same goes for HEPA vacuum cleaners. You are paying for HEPA vacuuming. How do you know the vacuums are really HEPA? You can't trust the label. Ask them to check the vacuums with the laser particle counter. Readings should be recorded in the logbook.

LOG BOOK for: _____ **(Address)**   **DATE:**
HEPA VACCUM AND NEG AIR FAN / SCRUBBER LASER PARTICLE COUNT READINGS

EQUIPMENT	Total particle counts 0.3 microns and larger		
	Ambient Air	Exhaust	% Reduction
Negative air fan / Air Scrubber #1			
Negative air fan / Air Scrubber # 2 (If applicable)			
HEPA Vacuum #1			
HEPA Vacuum #2			
% Reduction in particles = (Ambient – Exhaust reading) ÷ Ambient reading			
Comments:			

Sample logbook for recording laser particle count readings of HEPA vacuums and HEPA air scrubbers.

Day 2 - What to look for

After the containment is up, workers should remove anything that is in the way. This may be cabinets, toilets, bathtubs, and so forth depending on the room.

Next they should remove drywall, any rot, and sand or wire-brush the wood framing, exterior sheathing and roof decking as necessary. These activities should be done in a manner that minimizes dust and keeps the work area as clean as possible at all times. No spraying or fogging should be done. Antimicrobials should not be used.

Ask workers to show you pictures of mold as they remove drywall. This way you know if they are cutting too much or too little drywall out.

Out to Lunch

This was a large commercial project that took place in a shopping mall downtown. It cost tens of thousands of dollars. There was mold inside one of the stores.

We explained to the other stores that an exhaust duct from the negative air machine would run through the mall to get to the outside. We explained that the negative air pressure created would protect other shops from dust while the work was going on.

The workers had taped black plastic over the windows and were trying to keep things low-key. I was downtown for lunch and peeked my head in. I saw the air scrubber sitting in the middle of the store with no exhaust duct attached to it. The workers were afraid that if shoppers saw an exhaust duct going through the mall, there might be concern. The workers decided they would run the scrubber without exhausting it outside.

The workers used hammers, pounding on the ceiling to make the drywall come off. Drywall was falling to the floor in large clouds of dust. They should have been careful removing the mold. They were using push brooms to push all the moldy pieces into one big

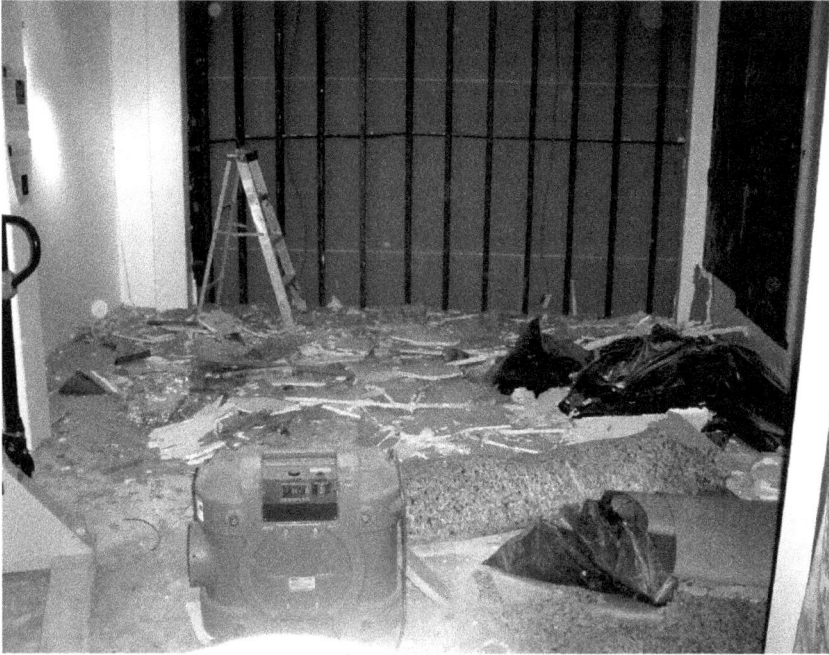

A big mess. This building owner did not get the specialized, technical work they paid for. Notice the air scrubber does not have an exhaust duct attached. There was an excessive amount of mold in the air because scraps of moldy drywall were lying around, drywall that was torn from the ceiling with hammers.

pile in the middle of the store. The mall was paying top dollar for HEPA vacuums, not push brooms. While this was going on I tested the air in the shops next door. The laboratory results showed *Stachybotrys* in the air.

Day 3

By the third day workers might be finished with demolition and start what is called the final cleaning. The final cleaning should be done with plain soap and water.

Before they tell you to call the mold inspector they should inspect their own work. If you feel comfortable, enter the containment and check that things are clean. Wear a respirator. Don't be intimidated by warning signs. There should be less or no mold. If the remediation tells you to stay out, that's a red flag.

The remediation company should shut the scrubber off before you call the mold inspector for a final test. The air scrubber needs to be off 24 hours before the mold inspector tests.

You, not the remediation company, should call the mold inspector. Having the mold remediation company hire the mold inspector is a conflict of interest because the mold inspector, wanting to get repeat business from the mold remediation company, may not be as strict in their inspection and testing as they would normally be.

You will note a line item on the estimate, "Equipment decontamination, per piece of equipment." Each air scrubber and vacuum cleaner is counted as a piece of equipment. Some power tools are counted. How they come up with the estimated number of hours and number of pieces of equipment is a mystery. Since you are being charged by the hour maybe you want to ask them to record how much time is dedicated to the task. Or maybe this is similar to going to a car dealership and being charged a shop fee. You just have to pay it. On a job, for example, with eight pieces of equipment, the cost of decontamination was $374. That's based on a line item rate of $40-50 dollars per piece of equipment. All they should be doing is wiping the equipment down with soap and water.

Once was not enough. Neither was twice.

This house had a roof leak that caused an interior wall to become wet. The wood framing inside the wall grew mold. I told the contractor to remove the drywall, sand or replace the wood framing, and call me to re-inspect.

He removed the drywall, cleaned the wood, rebuilt the wall and called me to do an inspection.

I could not do an inspection because the wall had been rebuilt. Therefore, I tested the wall again. The test results came back from the laboratory showing mold.

I explained that mold is microscopic and sometimes hard to see. I tried to communicate to the contractor that he has to be extra careful and methodical when cleaning. He went back to work, removing the new drywall and re-cleaning. He installed new drywall and called me to re-inspect.

Once again, I could not do a visual inspection because he had already installed new drywall. I re-tested the wall and the lab results came back with mold.

Contractors do not have the same definition of clean as some of us. Don't rebuild anything until the mold inspector can do a visual inspection.

Small Wonder

This is a case of mold that was in the ceiling of a small bathroom from a roof leak. I suggested they remove the entire bathroom ceiling. The estimator told the workers to remove only the middle part. It was a small bathroom. The job cost a few thousand dollars.

The workers, day labors, removed exactly what they were told by the supervisor and called me to test when they were done. I looked inside the hole they cut in the ceiling and saw mold. I told them to cut more of the ceiling out. They called their boss to get approval.

The supervisor insisted they had done a good job.

I talked to the owner of the company and told him I could see mold. He didn't believe me so he came over and looked. He agreed, handed the homeowner a work order change and charged more to remove more drywall from the ceiling. It would have been quicker if they had removed the entire ceiling to begin with. They also charged to re-clean the entire bathroom a second time, another double expense.

It's only Mold

This was a project in a large office building. Some of the walls and ceilings contained asbestos. An asbestos abatement company was hired to remove the asbestos and the mold. Asbestos remediation has been around longer than mold remediation so you would think an asbestos abatement company would know how to do things the correct way. I was surprised by the poor quality of work.

The remediator used duct tape to secure the exhaust duct to the air scrubber, the exhaust duct being vented outdoors. The exhaust duct fell off the air scrubber and blew air out into the hallway of the main office. The remediator did not remove both sides of the office walls. They removed one side of the walls and painted shellac over mold that was growing on the other side.

"We Do Mold All the Time"

I hear it frequently. Contractors who say they do mold all the time. Almost all do it wrong and they charge you as if they know what they are doing.

This case involved a leaky roof. The contractor cut the wall open, removed drywall and called me to do an inspection. I could see mushrooms growing near the ceiling on wood that was still wet.

I asked the contractor, "What are those?"

"Mushrooms?" he asked. He did not understand what clean meant. The plywood was rotten and needed to be removed. At the minimum he should have sanded the wood so it *looked* clean.

He called me the next day to say he was ready for another inspection. I found he had installed new drywall. I couldn't inspect the wood. He admitted to not replacing it. The homeowner didn't want to pay for me to do more testing. Chances are there are still mold and mushrooms in that wall today.

They knew there was (not) an easier way

This was a house a group of contractors purchased thinking they could flip it. The first time we meet I explained it was going to be a difficult job. Every wall in the house, every piece of framing and lumber, had mold on it. I suggested they use a sand-blaster to remove the mold.

They called me weeks later for an inspection. I found they had missed a lot of spots. There was visible mold throughout the house. I went home feeling bad for them.

A few weeks later I got another call.

"Come test," they said. "We have good air test results."

I returned and found things cleaner but could still see mold. They kept saying they have good air tests. It made me suspicious. I pried. They confessed they used a mold stain remover. The mold stain remover sealed the mold.

I said, "Yes, you have good air test results but there is still mold. You have to sand the wood because there is mold under the sealer."

They never called me back.

Key Points To Remember From Chapter 8

• You need to be watching.
• Make sure the containment is set up correctly with a negative air pressure created. The air scrubber (negative air machine) needs to be exhausted outside through a door or window.
• Ask the contractor to keep a logbook of activities and line items you will be charged for.

Chapter 9

ASK FOR A FINAL INVOICE BASED ON ACTUAL EXPENSES, NOT LINE ITEMS IN THE ESTIMATE

This part is tedious, technical and no fun. If you want to save money, this is how it's done.

Keep it simple. Go down the bill and look for big-ticket items: scrubber rental, antimicrobials (which should not have been used), filter changes, and so forth. Look for things that don't seem like they were done based on your observations.

If they charged you for a new HEPA filter (they did) ask them to verify that a new one was installed.

A good remediation company will show you their work sheets and log books.

Check the logbook to see how many times the pre-filters were changed on the air scrubber. It is reasonable to put a new pre-filter in the HEPA air scrubber at the start of the job and change the pre-filter before the final cleaning. If it's a dirty job they may change filters in between. That's a maximum total of twice (two pre-filter changes).

Check to see how many respirator cartridges were disposed of. It is reasonable to charge for respirator changes for every person for every day or second day. The reality is, some workers do not wear respirators or do not change the filters every day. Notice that there is a separate line item for workers wearing a respirator. The filter changes are in addition to them charging just to wear a respirator.

Check the worksheet. A good company will show you the measurements they took when the job was completed. Check how many square feet of walls were cut out, how many square feet of wood were wire-brushed and cleaned. To calculate the final bill, they should have taken the worksheet and put the actual number of square feet into the software that created the original estimate.

Measure the square footage of the work area. This affects the line item for detailed HEPA vacuuming and cleaning. If they made the work area smaller they didn't need to clean as much as estimated in their drawings.

If they replaced rotten wood (framing, exterior sheathing, or roof decking) you should not be paying to have it cleaned. The original estimate may have specified cleaning.

When it might cost *more* than an estimate

Almost all of the time, most of the mold is hiding. There's no way to know how much mold there is until you start opening walls or ceilings. Sometimes it might cost more than what is estimated. Most estimates are worst-case scenarios.

WORK SHEET for: _____ (Address)   **DATE:**

LINE ITEM COMMENT	SQFT	Linear Feet
SQFT Barrier / Airlock / Dcon Chamber		
Work Area (Containment) Walls (SQFT)		
Work Area (Containment) Floor (SQFT)		
Work Area (Containment)Ceiling (SQFT)		
Tear out Drywall (SQFT)		
Tear out Plaster (SQFT)		
Tear out Insulation (SQFT)		
Clean Studs (LF)		
Wire Brush, Sand, Scrape Walls (SQFT)		
Wire Brush, Sand, Scrape Floor (SQFT)		
Wire Brush, Sand, Scrape Exterior Sheathing (SQFT)		
Wire Brush, Sand, Scrape Roof Decking (SQFT)		
Baseboards (LF)		
Door Trim (LF)		

Sample worksheet. After the job is completed, the supervisor should take measurements of what was done. This should entered into the software that was used to create the estimate.

When it cost *exactly* the estimate

Some remediators stick to the estimate and blinders go on. The workers remove mold only from the area on the estimate. They spend their time (your money) HEPA vacuuming and cleaning only for the mold inspector to show up and find mold just outside the estimated area. You may be charged twice since they have to re-clean the entire room after they remove the mold they missed.

This could be avoided by making sure the mold remediator reads the mold inspector's report and uses common sense. Often the issue is that the workers are not supervised. They just do what they are told by the supervisor before he leaves them on their own.

Food for Thought

The most expensive part of mold remediation is containment (negative air machine, filter changes, plastic, and so forth). It's a reasonable cost to wire-brush and sand mold off wood. Wire brushing and sanding are quoted at less than one dollar per square foot.

As difficult as it sounds, it does not cost as much to remove cabinets and fixtures as it does to set up containment.

Something that can add up in cost is covering contents and fixtures and flooring with plastic. That's because of the large square footage. The price per square foot of plastic seems reasonable; often hundreds to thousands of square feet are involved.

Respirator cartridges cost as much as $24. If each worker changes them twice a day, four days, that's almost $400. If that's what it takes to protect workers, fine. The reality is, workers don't change their respirator cartridges that often; some do not wear them all of the time; some do not wear them at all.

The cost of the disposable suits can add up as well. One estimate had PPE suits changed 27 times over 3 days. At $17 each that came to $474. How many suits really went into the trash?

Final Thoughts

In the end I suppose it comes back to trust. You're either going to trust the company you hire or not. Maybe consider it charity towards their business if you pay for things that were not used, not done or unnecessary.

Hopefully you found a good remediation company and even if the line items don't seem accurate, the cost of having the job done right is worth it to you. Maybe you don't want to bother the remediation company with record keeping details. Maybe you want to consider yourself lucky you found someone who removed the mold properly and don't want to upset them by nitpicking at how they came up with the final bill.

Chapter 10

CONSIDER DOING IT YOURSELF

Can you do it yourself?

Sometimes you have to.

Take the Hernandez family. They live near a river that had a one in a hundred years flood. They didn't have flood insurance. They were smart enough to know that chemicals and bleach are not the answer.

With help from thirty family members and community volunteers, they pulled out every cabinet in the house and tore drywall out to two feet high. They squeegeed the water out the front door and wet vacuumed the rest. They rented dehumidifiers and carpet fans to accelerate drying. During the day they opened windows and burned wood in the fireplace. They found a thirty-dollar moisture meter at the hardware store and monitored how the drying was going. They were trying to dry things to zero percent moisture. When I meet them I explained that wood absorbs moisture from the air; ten percent is considered dry.

I came to do a mold inspection two weeks after the flood. There was some dried mud on the floor but no mold except for one small spot underneath one cabinet. They did a better job of drying things and removing any mold that grew than most professionals.

Before worrying too much...

No matter how much you or your contractor screw up, odds are you are doing as good or better job than most professionals. When I am working with a mold remediation company that I have not worked with before, I usually find mold they have missed. They blame me for finding it and complain they never have this problem with other inspectors.

If you purchase an air scrubber and make sure it's setup the correct way (to create a negative air pressure) and the contractor uses soap and water instead of antimicrobials for cleaning, there can be no harm done.

Tools Required

Air scrubber. Buy one. You can sell it on e-bay.
HEPA vacuum. Buy one or use the best vacuum you can find.
Full-face respirator, disposable suits, gloves
Polyethylene sheeting and duct tape

Contractor grade trash bags
Razor blade, drywall saw, pry-bar
Wire brush
Dish soap, pail of water, rags

Trades Required

In addition to a plumber, roofer or other applicable trades
to make repairs to the source of moisture:

A General Contractor you can trust
A Certified Microbial Consultant (mold inspector)
Someone good at meticulously wire-brushing
A cleaning crew

The Process

Seal off the work area from the rest of the house with plastic, hung floor to ceiling. (If it's an entire room just close the door.) Place the air scrubber in the work area and run the exhaust duct from the scrubber to outside through a window.

Hire a mold inspector to check things *before* the contractor begins working. This also allows the opportunity for the consultant to discuss with the general contractor how mold is supposed to be removed.

Ask the general contractor to charge their regular rate. Tell them they are not being asked to do any kind of special work. The general contractor should do the demolition, tearing out walls and cutting out rot. He should remove cabinets and fixtures as necessary to remove any drywall that is affected behind them. Tell the contractor to remove drywall two feet past where he sees staining or mold on the backside. He should pull out insulation and cut out any rot (any rot on framing, sill plates, exterior sheathing, roof decking) as necessary. Contractors are good (and fast) at tearing things out. Since there will be a lot of dust generated, remind the contractor to occasionally change the pre-filters on the air scrubber.

Find someone else to do the detailed wire brushing and cleaning of the exposed wood. This is a critical step and the hardest to fulfill. It can be difficult to find someone who knows what clean means, someone who methodically uses the wire brush to clean the exposed framing, flooring, bottom of roof decking, exterior plywood sheathing and so forth. Give them the HEPA vacuum. They need to clean every stud and piece of framing with soap and water after it's wire-brushed. Keep the negative air pressure going.

Hire a specialized cleaning crew to do the final cleaning. Consider a post-construction cleaning service that does the clean up on construction sites.

Call the mold inspector back to do a final inspection and testing.

All of this should be easy to coordinate except the step of wire brushing. It might be difficult to find someone good at wire-brushing mold off wood framing. This process is not bullet proof. Otherwise I would recommend it to everyone.

Resources

The following are provided for those who might do the work themselves or hire a general contractor to help.

Personal Protective Equipment (PPE)

I have an on-line course that covers what to wear to stay safe while doing mold remediation. Register at www.academy.healthylivingspaces.com. The course is free to readers. At checkout use the coupon code MOLDMONEY to receive 100% off.

Full-face respirators and disposable suits

I wear the following:
• Kimberly Clark KleenGuard A40 Coveralls
• A Honeywell North 7600 Full-Face Respirator

Filters for respirators are sold separately. If there are odors, the combination cartridge/filter, Organic Vapor (OV)/P100 is suggested. If only mold particles are a concern, P100 filters suffice. Supplies can be found at:

Grainger.com
1-800-GRAINGER

Air Scrubbers

650 CFM is the minimum air flow suggested. I've seen air scrubbers/negative air machines that appear to cost less. If you read the specs you must buy several and hook them together to achieve the stated CFM and the HEPA filter is thin. You don't need carbon.

Abatement Technologies

For small jobs, the PAS750 (750 CFM) is sufficient. You'll need to a box of flexible ducting, a clamp to connect the duct to the machine, and a box of each type of pre-filter (coarse and fine). A new machine comes with a HEPA filter installed. You won't need to change it.
Phone: (800) 634-9091
www.abatement.com

Aerospace America

Metal, 3-stage, high-CFM units for a good price.
Phone: (800) 237-6414
www.aerospaceamerica.com

Dri-Eaz®

These are popular with remediation companies. They are made with plastic and have only two stages of filtration: a MERV 8 pre-filter and HEPA.

HEPA Vacuums

I use a Nilfisk Model GM80. There are larger models that may be more appropriate for big, messier jobs.
www.nilfisk.com

Part 4

How to Prevent Mold from Reoccurring

Antimicrobials are not the answer

Water it and they will grow. You've got to get rid of the water. Fix the plumbing leak. Repair the roof. Solve the moisture problem. Contact a professional if you need help identifying the source. We call this a moisture investigation.

Use the garden hose

If the source of moisture is an outside leak, before you rebuild the walls, identify where the leak is and make sure it has been fixed. A good tool is the garden hose. If a window is what was leaking and it's been fixed, go outside and hose down the window while someone inside watches for water to come in. Be prepared to stop if water comes in. It helps to have a thermal imaging camera and moisture meter to spot small leaks.

If it's a roof leak, put the hose on the roof and let it run while someone inside watches for leaks.

Here's an example where Mother Nature had the garden hose. A remediation company cut drywall out under a window and called me to inspect. As I was finishing, a fast moving monsoon blew though. Water immediately dripped inside under the window. There was a small crack along the bottom of the window outside. The window was on the second story. Nobody had gone up on a ladder to check.

DenseGlass®

If not for paper we wouldn't have so many mold problems. Even the Three Pigs didn't build their houses out of paper.

That's what is on both sides of conventional drywall.

There is a better way - fiberglass on the front and backsides instead of paper. It's called *DensArmor® Interior Wallboard* or DensGlass® Sheathing. Mold can't eat fiberglass.

Use it in places that might become wet (around bathrooms and kitchens). Install it on exterior walls. Why not use it everywhere? It's almost the same price as conventional drywall. Commercial builders took to it right away. It's the yellow board you see on large office buildings under construction. (Just think how many older commercial building have mold because they were built with paper-faced drywall).

Green board, a type of wallboard installed around showers, is made with paper. It is treated and resistant to mold but mold will eventually grow on it.

When installing any kind of drywall, leave a 1/4" gap off the bottom of the floor. This prevents water from wicking up the wall in the event there is a flood.

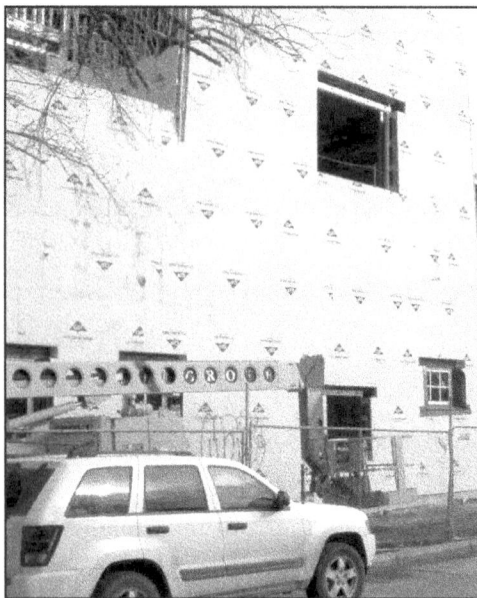

DensGlass® on the exterior of a commercial building.

SUGGESTED READING

ANSI/IICRC S520 Standard for Professional Mold Remediation, Institute of Inspection, Cleaning and Restoration Certification (IICRC).

Guidelines on Assessment and Remediation of Fungi in Indoor Environments, New York City Department of Health.

Damp Indoor Spaces and Health, Institute of Medicine of the National Academies, The National Academies Press, Washington, D.C.

IICRC S500 Standard and Reference Guide for Professional Water Damage Restoration, Institute of Inspection, Cleaning and Restoration (IICRC).

Appendix 1

Sample Mold Remediation Protocol

IMPORTANT NOTICE

The following is a SUMMARY, a SIMPLIFIED VERSION of what should be provided in a mold remediation protocol written by a Microbial Consultant (CMC). The intention is to provide a sample for those unable to hire a consultant to write a customized one. The information contained here is not intended to be the sole instructions used by a homeowner, contractor or mold remediation company to facilitate the execution of the steps herein.

Contact Healthy Living Spaces for detailed specifications for your project, (505) 603-8101.

Mold Remediation Protocol for Mold Remediation to be performed at

_____

(Address)

Appropriate Standards and Guidelines will be followed

The removal of water damaged and microbial contaminated building materials and cleaning of exposed surfaces shall be done according to the _IICRC S520 Standard for Professional Mold Remediation._

Notice regarding the use of anything other than plain soap and water

No chemicals or cleaning products may be used other than fragrance-free dish-soap and water.

This includes but is not limited to: stain removers, mold killers, mold control products, bleach, disinfectants, antimicrobials, biocides, deodorizers, anti-fungal treatments; products containing ammonia, alcohol, petroleum; products with the words: Warning, Hazardous, Caution, and Harmful. This includes ozone and essential oils. It includes products with EPA registrations.

Containment

It is the contractor's responsibility to ensure that containment with negative air pressure and all other steps are taken to prevent cross-contamination of dust inside the work area to areas outside the work area.

Negative Air Pressure

One or more HEPA-filtered, negative air machines (also know as air scrubbers) shall be used to maintain a negative pressure of 0.02 inches of water column (5 Pascal) in each work area with reference to the rest of the building and a minimum of four air exchanges per hour.

At the start of the job, a supervisor shall check the integrity of each HEPA air machine with a laser particle counter by measuring the exhaust compared to the ambient room air. There should be at least a 99% reduction in particle counts at the exhaust of the air machine compared to readings at the intake. For reference see the *Portable High Efficiency Air Filtration Device Field Testing and Validation* ("PHEAF") Standard developed by the Indoor Environmental Standard's Organization (IESO).

Air scrubbers shall be exhausted outside via ducts connected to scrubbers that go out a door or window.

An air scrubber shall never be used in re-circulation mode (where the scrubber exhaust is not vented outdoors).

Under no circumstances will an air scrubber/negative air machine be vented into another room of the building.

HEPA Vacuums

At the start of the job, a supervisor shall check the integrity of the HEPA vacuum by measuring the exhaust of the vacuum using a laser particle counter. There should be a 99% reduction in particle counts at the exhaust compared to ambient air readings.

Asbestos and Lead Paint

Buildings constructed before 1977 and as late as 1983 may contain asbestos.

Buildings constructed before 1960 and as late as 1978 may contain lead-based paint.

The contractor is responsible for making sure any building materials that will be disturbed do not contain asbestos or lead-based paint. The contractor will ask the client to have any suspect materials tested prior to disturbing them and if necessary, to contract a licensed abatement company to remove any identified hazardous materials.

Removal of Materials

Materials will be removed so as not to excessively agitate them and unnecessarily create dust:

• Do not use a hammer to demolish drywall.
• Unscrew or carefully pry gypsum board away from studs.
• Use razor knives.
• If a saw is used, set the saw blade such that the blade does not penetrate all the way through and finish removal by scoring the backing with a razor.
• Electric saws should have dust collection devices.
• Do not use any methods that would raise dust such as dry sweeping or vacuuming with equipment not equipped with HEPA filtration.

All porous materials (drywall and plaster for example) that are water damaged (stained, bubbled) or visibly contaminated with mold shall be removed two feet past locations from which mold and/or water damage appears to be visible on either the front or back sides. This may require the removal of cabinets, vanities, tubs, showers, etc. to facilitate.

Where water damage or mold originates from the ceiling or the top of the wall, drywall shall be removed floor to ceiling.

On interior walls, where water damage or mold is visible on one side of a wall, the drywall on the other side of the wall shall also be removed to the same height.

Drywall, insulation and other materials that are removed shall immediately be placed in 6 mil plastic bags. Debris shall not be allowed to accumulate in a pile on the floor. The work area is to be kept as clean and free of debris as possible.

Exposed insulation should be removed and discarded.

Rot should be removed. This includes any applicable sill plates, framing, exterior sheathing, roof decking, etc.

Semi-porous materials such as wood that are not removed will be restored and cleaned by mechanical means (wire-brushing or sanding) until clean and free of both mold and staining. This includes any sill plates, framing, exterior sheathing, roof decking, etc.

Final Cleaning
This should be done with the air scrubber running with negative air pressure.

Using HEPA vacuums, vacuum floors, inside wall cavities, corner pockets of the wall framing to remove the bulk of settled dust and debris.

Use a compressed air hose to blow dust from the insides of wall cavities and hard to reach areas. Allow the dust to settle then re-vacuum. Repeat until the structure appears to be clean of larger debris and there is not a noticeable amount of dust blowing out of interstitial spaces.

Do a final HEPA vacuum of all surfaces, top to bottom, floor to ceiling.

Damp-wipe all surfaces using soap and water. Work from top to bottom. Include ceilings, framing, surfaces inside exposed wall and ceiling cavities, walls and floors. Clean rags should be folded in quarters and dipped into the cleaning solution (plain soap and water). The rags shall be wrung out to remove excess moisture. The wiping surface shall be changed after each pass across a material. Rags may not re-enter the cleaning solution. Exhausted rags should be disposed.

Post Remediation Verification (Clearance) Testing

The *remediation company* shall perform a post-remediation evaluation prior to contacting the mold inspector to do post testing (Section 12.2.11 of the *S520*). The evaluation shall ensure surfaces are visually clean, free of odors and dry.

When, based on their post-remediation evaluation, the remediator feels confident they have removed all the mold, they shall call the Microbial Consultant to perform a final inspection and testing.

The contractor shall shut the air scrubber(s) off a minimum of twenty-four hours before the mold inspector performs testing.

Plastic used for containment shall remain in place until after satisfactory test results are obtained from the laboratory.

Rebuilding should not occur until after the inspection and testing indicates a clean environment.

If the samples pass the criteria established by the Microbial Consultant, regular construction personnel can enter the work area to do reconstruction.

It is recommended that containment (plastic sheeting and the air scrubber running to create a negative air pressure) remain in place during re-construction to capture dust generated during re-construction activities.

Record Keeping
The remediation company shall keep a logbook / worksheet on site that documents:

• Laser particle measurements used to verify the integrity of the air scrubber / negative air machine(s) and HEPA vacuums
• The air pressure differential between the containment and outside the containment
• The name and date of the worker performing the post-remediation evaluation with a statement of their findings and recommendations and that the job is ready to call the mold inspector to do the final inspector and testing.

STUDIES ON PRODUCTS USED
TO KILL MOLD

This section provides studies performed by Healthy Living Spaces (HLS) in partnership with Los Alamos National Laboratories (LANL). For two years HLS and LANL studied products used to treat mold. Our intention was to evaluate how well these products killed mold.

It should be understood that the purpose of these studies was not to focus on certain products or groups of products. You will note that the brand names were omitted in the first studies. The products in the second experiments are different than those in the first. The lesson is that products used to treat mold or remove mold stains, products used to kill mold, even some that say they remove mold, do not behave strictly as labeled.

During our experiments it was observed that some products encapsulate mold, even those not labeled to do so. We found products encapsulate mold in a fashion that makes it difficult for the home inspector to detect mold afterwards. Some of our final studies were efforts to devise new test methods for mold inspectors to use, tests to tell if a house was treated for mold. If it were discovered that a house was treated, one could be extra careful during inspections to check for mold that may have been treated instead of removed.

We started to evaluate what compounds and chemicals may reside after using products. That work is unfinished.

A study to evaluate the effectiveness of products used to kill mold or remove mold stains and if their use alters the effectiveness of using surface samples (tape-lifts) to detect residual mold

By Daniel Stih and Kirk D. Rector

Daniel Stih
Healthy Living Spaces
369 Montezuma Ave #169
Santa Fe, New Mexico 87501

Kirk D. Rector
Chemistry Division
Los Alamos National Laboratory
Los Alamos, NM 87567

Corresponding Author: (505) 603-8101
email: dan@healthylivingspaces.com

Keywords: *mold, surface samples, tape lift, swab, fungal spores, fungi, anti- microbial, hydrogen peroxide*

ABSTRACT

This paper describes an experiment that was performed to evaluate if the use of products sold as mold killers and mold stain removers may inhibit the effectiveness of surface samples (tape-lifts) to detect residual mold after these products have been applied. Surface samples (tape-lifts) are routinely used by consultants (mold inspectors) to verify the effectiveness of mold remediation projects. Surface samples are used to verify surfaces are clean and do not contain mold growth. A mold contaminated utility closet in a home was used. Products were applied to keep surfaces wet for at least ten minutes. Surface samples were taken before treatment, six hours after treatment, and twenty-four hours after treatment.

Based on an analysis of surface samples collected (tape-lifts), the conclusion is that products alone do not remove all of the mold growth present and that the use of products may inhibit the detection of the residual mold. The products appear to encapsulate the surfaces altering the way spores normally transfer to tape lifts. Use of products may make it difficult to use tape lifts as they are traditionally used to test for mold after remediation is completed. Using tape lifts (surface samples) may lead to the false conclusion that mold has been removed when it has not been.

I. Introduction

Traditionally, mold remediation was performed by removing mold versus trying to treat or kill it. The New York City Department of Health was one of the first public health organizations to provide guidance on how to remediate mold. Created in 2000, much of the information contained in *Guidelines on Assessment and Remediation of Fungi in Indoor Environments* was subsequently adopted by the EPA (1). According to these Guidelines, porous materials (wall board) should be removed and discarded. Cleaning should be performed using soap or a detergent solution using the gentlest cleaning method that effectively removes the mold. Disinfectants are seldom needed because the removal of fungal growth remains the most effective way to prevent exposure. The use of gaseous or aerosolized (fogging) biocides is not recommended (1).

Most professional mold remediators are familiar with the *IICRC S520 Standard for Professional Mold Remediation* (2). It is an ANSI standard that has been peer reviewed and is widely accepted and recognized in the industry. According to the *S520*, removal of mold contamination should always be the primary means of remediation. Indiscriminate use of antimicrobials, coatings, sealants and cleaning chemicals is not recommended. Porous material (drywall) should be removed and discarded. Semi-porous materials such as wood should be cleaned by mechanical means (wire-brushing or sanding).

Removing mold is more expensive and time consuming than treating it. There are now products on the market that suggest they can be used to provide a quick turnaround time without the need for demolition and removing the materials contaminated with mold or cleaning them by sanding or wire-brushing. This paper will study if they work (remove the mold). This paper will study if the use of these products may inhibit the detection of any residual mold these products do not remove.

Traditionally, after a mold remediation project is completed, a consultant independent of the contractor performing the remediation work, tests to verify that the mold has been removed. This testing may consist of a combination of surface and/or air sampling. Surface samples are typically taken to ensure that the readily accessible surfaces are clean and clean of any actual mold growth. Tape-lift samples are the preferred way of taking surface samples (*vs.* a swab) as there is direct transfer of the particles and mold from the surfaces to the tape. Residual particle matter and mold can be observed under the microscope without the need to culture. Using a swab can damage the structure of the mold mycelium and spores present.

If products used to treat mold leave residuals or coatings, it may be difficult to obtain reliable surface lift samples. There is the potential that any spores and particles present on the surface will not transfer to the tape. The significance of this is that the consultant doing the testing may conclude that the mold has been removed when it has not.

II. Methods & Materials

Types of Mold Killers and Mold Stain Removers Evaluated
The first product evaluated (Product 1) is sold as a mold stain re-

mover. It is sold in a package of two bottles, one that contains a dry power substance; one that is a liquid. The two bottles are mixed together by adding them to water and applied using a spray bottle or by fogging. According to the manufacturer, the product can be used as an alternative to sanding or wire-brushing mold off surfaces. According to the Material Safety Data Sheet (MSDS), the bottles for Product 1 contain arylesterase (<1%), propylene glycol diacetate (48-52%), and sodium percarbonate (47-51%). According to the MSDS, when mixed with water the product forms peracetic acid (most likely by the oxidation of the acetaldehyde).

The EPA first registered peracetic acid as an antimicrobial in 1985 for use on hard surfaces. As an oxidizing agent, sodium percarbonate is an ingredient in a number of laundry cleaning products. Dissolved in water, it yields a mixture of hydrogen peroxide and sodium carbonate. Sodium carbonate, sold as washing soda, can be used to remove grease, oil and stains and as a descaling agent. Propylene glycol diacetate is typically used as a solvent or plasticizer. It hydrolyses to acetic acid and propylene glycol when mixed with water. The manufacturer did not disclose what the purpose of the propylene glycol is in the mold stain remover product but possible reasons include to increase the overall viscosity of the spray or to expand the temperature range that the treatment is active over.

The second product (Product 2) evaluated is a hydrogen peroxide based formula. There are two equal parts liquid that are mixed together prior to use. It can be applied by sprayer or by fogging. Product literature says it kills mold on contact and requires no invasive demolition. According to the MSDS, the product contains quaternary ammonium compounds (1.6%), hydrogen peroxide (3.98%; 1 ppm) and inert ingredients (94.42%). The exact type of quaternary ammonium compounds is not listed although these generally act by disrupting cell membranes. It should be noted that the term "inert" does not mean non-toxic. While in chemistry the term "inert" is used to describe a substance that is not chemically reactive, for antimicrobials registered with the EPA, the term is defined by the federal law that governs pesticides: Federal Insecticide, Fungicide, and Rodenticide Act (FIFRA). According to FIFRA, where as an active ingredient is one that prevents, destroys, repels, or mitigates a pest, all other ingredients are called inert ingredients. Examples include those that related to foaming, extending product shelf life, solvents used to penetrate, and ingredients that generally used to increase the effectiveness of the active ingredients.

The third product evaluated is a 3% solution of hydrogen peroxide obtained at a local drug store.

Experiment Methods

A moldy mechanical room in a residential home was used for this experiment. The back interior wall was covered with mold to a height of approximately five feet. Conditions were dry at the time of testing. The water was shut off. Plastic sheeting was used to partition the back wall into two segments that are isolated from each other. Product 1 was sprayed on the left side (next to the right side of the hot water heater); Product 2 was sprayed on the right side of the partition (the left side of the boiler and behind the boiler); the drug store 3% hydrogen peroxide was sprayed on the wall in front of the platform. Images are shown in Figure 1.

The products were mixed and prepared according to instructions on the labels. Surfaces were sprayed so that surfaces remained wet for at least ten minutes. Surfaces were measured with a moisture meter and found to be damp (20%) six hours later. Surface samples were collected before and twenty-four hours after the application of products. It should be understood that the use of tape to obtain a surface sample removes some of the mold present on a surface where the tape is applied. As best possible, tape lifts taken after the application of the products were taken nearby but not exactly in the same location. Colored pushpins were used to note the areas where surface samples were taken before applying products.

III. Results and Discussion

Macroscopically, there is visible mold and staining present after the application for all the products tested. The surfaces treated with Product 1 and Product 2 seemed to be less dark, less black than before treatment, probably from the oxidation process. The surfaces treated with drug store 3% hydrogen peroxide did not appear to change color or contrast. In collecting surface samples from surfaces treated with Product 1 and Product 2, these products seemed to leave a microscopic coating on the surface of the drywall. For many of the samples collected from the surfaces treated with Product 1 and Product 2, it was necessary to remove a portion of the drywall paper onto the tape to transfer the darker (mold) particles onto the tape. This was not the case for samples collected from surfaces treated with drug store 3% hydrogen peroxide. The mold particles on those surfaces appeared to readily transfer to the tape, similar to how they did before treating the surface.

The tape samples were studied using an Olympus LEXT4000 3D optical scanning microscope. The use of this instrument gives a benefit of acquiring both high spatial resolution and true color information. Another benefit is that 3D scans are acquired from which extended focus images are generated. This acquisition strategy enables large areas to be acquired in focus. This last benefit is important for tape liftoffs where material embedded into the adhesive can be at different depths than the focus depth of high numerical aperture objectives.

Figure 5 shows tape-lift sample collected in region 1 prior to treatment with product 1. Individual *Stachybotrys* spores, small clusters of spores, and some hyphae are visualized. Figure 5 show similar areas after treatment. In both cases, there is significant aggregation of spores into clusters, as well as colorization with some regions appearing red or brown unseen in the prior treatment sample. The spores appear opaque instead of dark colored probably because they were oxidized (bleached) by the treatment. The hyphae appear to be destroyed and no longer tubular appearing. In the aggregated regions the outlines of the spores can be visualized and material between the spores is also seen.

Figure 6 shows similar results to Figure 5 with darker, redder appearance and apparently destroyed hyphae. One distinction between Figure 5 and 6 are that Figure 6 appears to show individual spores encapsulated with material making them bigger by 2-4x.

Figures 7 are microphotographs of surface samples (tape-lifts) collected from the area in front of the platform before and after treatment with drug store 3% hydrogen peroxide. In figure 7 before treatment, *Stachybotrys* is readily visible, as also seen in figures 6 and 5. Figure 7 shows the similar area acquired 24 hours after treatment. There does not appear to be any reduction in the number of spores or significant change in the spore structure (absence/presence of mycelium) or color compared to microphotographs taken of surface sample before treatment with 3% hydrogen peroxide.

In addition to macroscopic and microscopic imagery, similar to how tape lift samples were collected, swab samples were taken before and twenty-four hours after treatments. The swab samples were cultured for viable fungi using Malt Extract Agar (MEA) and Cellulose based agar. The culture results were different depending on what type of media used. MEA is generally used for the isolation of broad-spectrum fungi; while cellulose based agar is used specifically to isolate *Stachybotrys*. The swab samples were cultured and analyzed by an independent laboratory.

Table I and Table II show the results for cultures of samples collected before and after the surfaces were treated in cellulose and MEA, respectively. The results are expressed in colony forming units (CFU) per swab. Each sampled area was approximately one square inch. Only the types of mold that were detected are listed.

It seems there was nearly a 100% reduction in the viability of spores treated with Product 2. There did not seem to be as much of a reduction in the viability of spores for surfaces treated with Product 1 or the 3% hydrogen peroxide. For the surfaces treated with 3% hydrogen peroxide there was a significant amount of *Stachybotrys* in both the before and after samples cultured using Cellulose agar (for *Stachybotrys*). However, the samples cultured using MEA agar showed an increase in yeasts. The reason for this is unknown. One possibility is if the bulk of *Stachybotrys* spores were rendered nonviable by the treatment, the yeast was able to thrive in the culture due to the lack of competing organisms. This is one of the reasons both the S520 and classic texts caution against using antimicrobials and biocides. Specifically, "Biocides and antimicrobial agents may show promise in laboratory test, but safe and effective use in building environments may be difficult. Some agents are designed to treat certain groups of microorganisms. However, suppression of one organism may give others an advantage, leading to different control problems (7)." Another words, when certain organisms are killed, an advantage is given to the surviving ones.

Viability studies present interesting results; however is not the complete picture with regard to mold removal. According to the EPA, "Mold spores and fragments can produce allergic reactions in sensitive individuals regardless of whether the mold is dead or alive (6)." Therefore, even if there is a reduction in the viability of any residual spores, there may not necessarily be a reduction in the health effects and symptoms associated with mold exposure unless the mold is physically removed.

IV. Conclusions

It is important to understand that this report is not comparing how brands of mold killers and mold stain removers perform relative to each other. What is being studied is how these products may affect tape lift sample results and if they actually remove mold and stains or just appear to encapsulate them. While it might seem interesting to compare how many spores may have been killed by each product, the first question to consider is: does the use of products eliminate mold such that the traditional methods of removing mold does not need to be followed?

Herein, it is concluded that none of the products tested completely eliminated the mold or staining present macroscopically. The use of products other than the 3% drug store hydrogen peroxide appears to encapsulate the surface with a clear, microscopic coating. The coating appears to inhibit the transfer of particles to tape lift samples. If one is not aggressive in collecting the tape samples (pressing hard and removing part of the paper backing of the drywall), mold may remain on the surface and not be transferred to the tape. Particles that are collected on the tape may be obscured by the presence of the paper from the drywall. This could prevent an analyst from observing any residual mold that may be present depending on how carefully the tape lifts are examined and how much particles are actually transferred to the tape.

The use of drug store 3% hydrogen peroxide did not appear to affect how particles are transferred to tape. Surface samples appeared the same before and after the application of the hydrogen peroxide although there might appear to be a slight browning effect on the spores. The use of hydrogen peroxide also does not appear to reduce the viability of mold spores. It is possible that the use of hydrogen peroxide may help clean up and sterilize surfaces from non-fungal matter (bacteria, allergens, etc.)

Use of these products may inhibit accurate testing results since while the mold does not appear to be removed it is not as readily observed with tape lifts. The trouble with using commercial products is that Products leave a residual and not all the ingredients are listed. Most manufacturers admit that products leave a residual antimicrobial, the exact type of which is not always disclosed. It is recommended that if users wish to have products other than hydrogen peroxide applied, they should only be applied after testing is performed and tests results indicate there is not mold growth on the surfaces.

V. Acknowledgements

Surface samples were analyzed by direct microscopic examination by Healthy Living Spaces LLC and Los Alamos National Laboratories (LANL). Healthy Living Spaces is a participant is LANL's Technical Assistance program.

VI. References

1. New York City Department of Health, *Guidelines on Assessment and Remediation of Fungi in Indoor Environments*, 2008.

2. Institute of Inspection, Cleaning and Restoration Certification (IICRC), *Standard and Reference Guide for Professional Mold Remediation*, (ANSI/IICRC S520-2008), Vancouver, WA, 2008.

3. Institute of Inspection, Cleaning and Restoration Certification (IICRC), *Standard and Reference Guide for Professional Mold Remediation,* (ANSI/IICRC S520-2008), Vancouver, WA, 2008, p.21

4. Institute of Inspection, Cleaning and Restoration Certification (IICRC), *Standard and Reference Guide for Professional Mold Remediation* (ANSI/IICRC S520-2008), Vancouver, WA, 2008.

5. "Inert Ingredients Frequently Asked Questions," United States Environmental Protection Agency, Office of Chemical Safety and Pollution Prevention, [Online] available at http://www.epa.gov/op-prd001/inerts/faqs.pdf (Accessed January 22, 2014).

6. "Mold Remediation in Schools and Commercial Buildings, Appendix B - Introduction to Molds," United States Environmental Protection Agency [Online] Available at http://www.epa.gov/mold/mold_remediation.html#append_b (Accessed January 22, 2014).

7. Janet Macher, Ed.: *Bioaerosols: Assessment and Control*, American Conference of Governmental Industrial Hygienists, 1999. Section 16.1.

Figure 1: Photos of site before treatment

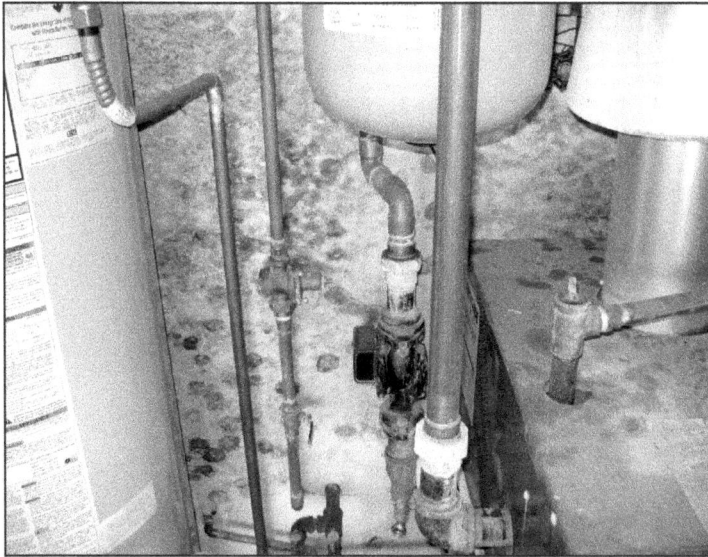

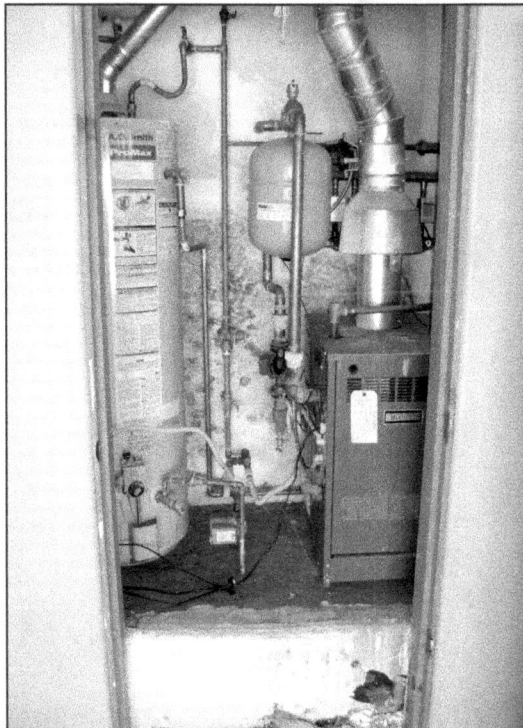

Figure 2A: Before treatment with Product 1

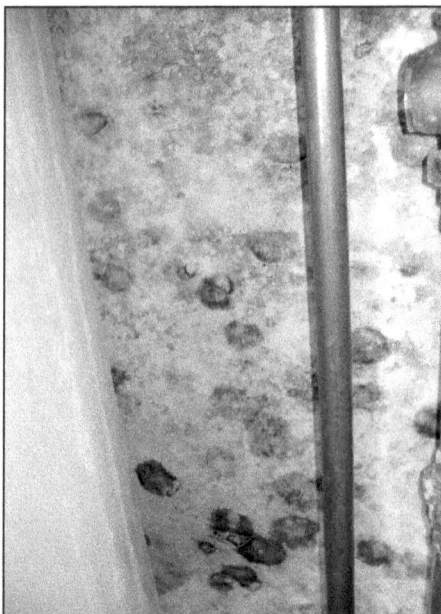

Figure 2B: 24 hours after treatment with Product 1

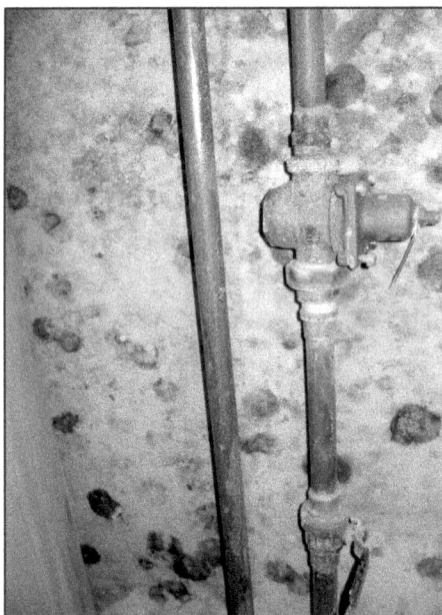

Figure 3A: Before treatment with Product 2

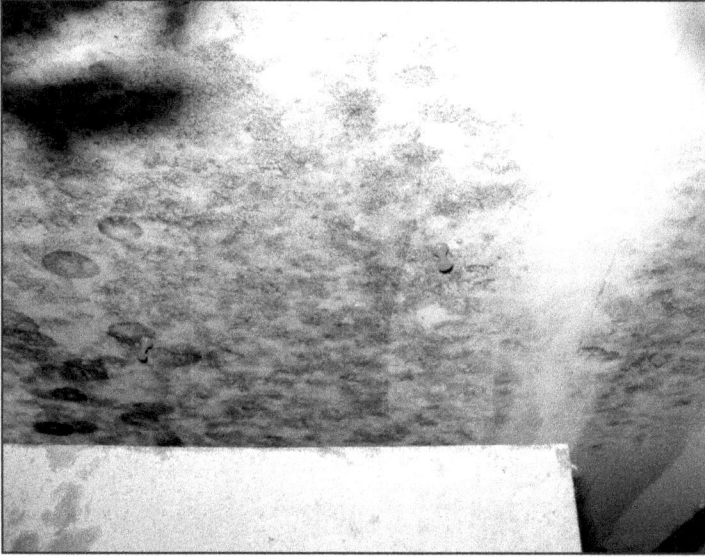

Figure 3B: 24 hours after treatment with Product 2

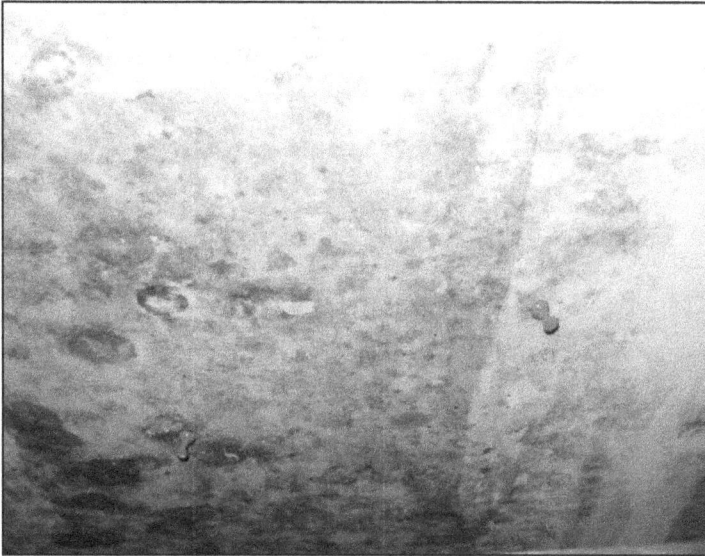

Figure 4A: Before treatment with 3% H2O2

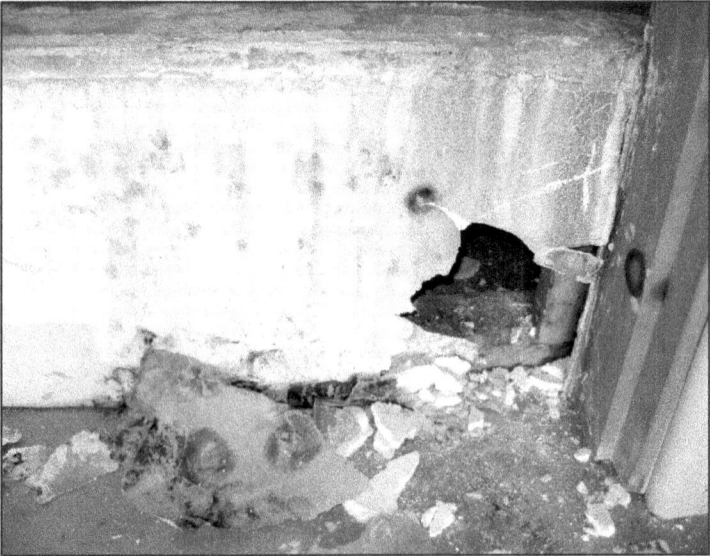

Figure 4B: 24 hours after treatment with 3% H2O2

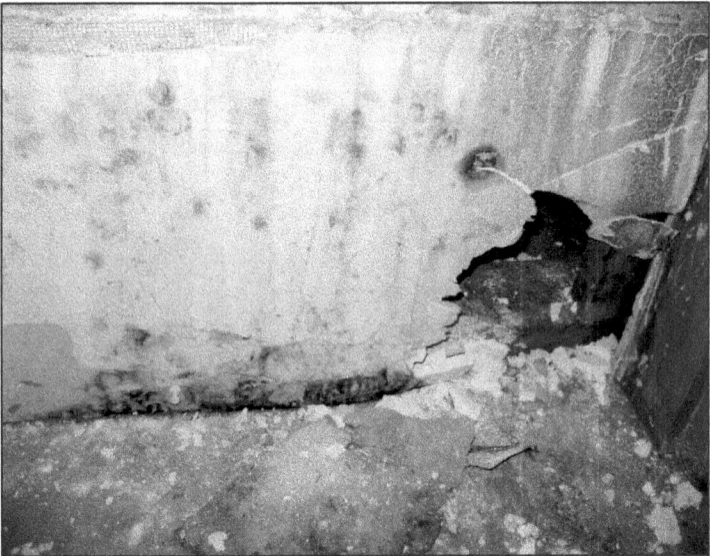

Figure 5: Tape-lift collected from area to be treated with Product 1 before treatment (left); after 6 hours post treatment (middle) and 24 hours post treatment (right). Scale bars are 40 microns.

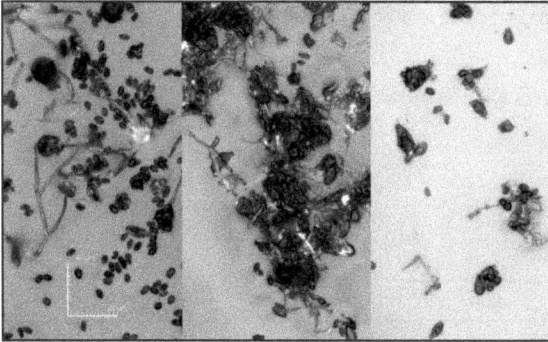

Figure 6: Tape-lift collected from area to be treated with Product 2 before treatment (left); after 6 hours post treatment (middle) and 24 hours post treatment (right). Scale bars are 40 microns.

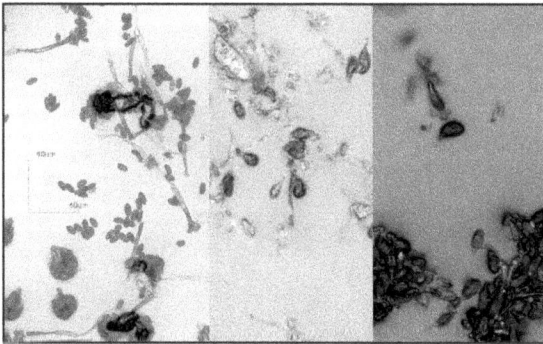

Figure 7: Tape-lift collected from area to be treated with 3% H2O2 before treatment (left); a 6 hours post treatment (middle) and 24 hours post treatment (right). Scale bars are 40 microns.

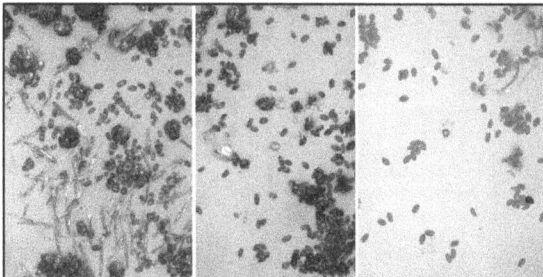

TABLE I. Viability of spores before and after treatments. Surface swabs cultured using Cellulose Agar. Surface areas approximately one square inch.

Colony Forming Units (CFU) per swab

	Product I		Product 2		3% Hydrogen Peroxide	
	Before	After	Before	After	Before	After
Penicillium		300	10,000			
Stachybotrys	110,000	1,000	170,000		540,000	770,000
Ulocladium		600	10,000			
Total	110,000	2,300	200,000	ND	540,000	770,000

TABLE II. Viability of spores before and after treatments. Surface swabs cultured using Malt Extract Agar (MEA). Surface areas approximately one square inch.

Colony Forming Units (CFU) per swab

	Product 1		Product 2		3% Hydrogen Peroxide	
	Before	After	Before	After	Before	After
Alternaria	3,000	10,000	22,000			10
Cladosporium	4,700		10,000			
Penicillium		70,000	37,000			310
Stachybotrys					680,000	
Yeasts		300,000				3,000
Total	7,700	470,000	75,000	10	680,000	3,300

Statement of Work

Understanding and detecting the use of products used to treat mold

For

Healthy Living Spaces

Company Background: Healthy Living Spaces LLC performs testing and investigations of residential and commercial building regarding building-related health complaints or concerns related to, but not limited to, toxic mold, dust, allergens, chemicals, odors and other indoor air quality/environmental quality pollutants.

Technical Assistance Requested:
1) Chemical Analysis of decontamination products
2) Analysis of samples treated with various decontamination products using advanced microscopy techniques
3) Analysis of samples subjected to accelerated aging for testing of stability of protective coating
4) Proposed mechanisms for testing for these products in the field

Project Goals: (As time and funds permit)
The primary objective here is to understand these products better. The results of such a study would answer questions such as:
How can a mold inspector know if these products were used (something that is currently quite difficult);
Can the residuals effect air or environmental quality;
How do the coatings these products leave hold up with age, temperature, humidity, etc;
The project may require providing some of the products to LANL and/or samples of surfaces treated with them.

Project Results & Deliverables:
LANL will supply a written report to company which summarizing results discovered during the project.

LANL Contact: Kirk Rector, C-PCS, MS J567, Tel: 505-667-9457, kdr@lanl.gov

Company Contact: Daniel Stih, 359 Montezuma Ave., Santa Fe, NM 87501,Tel: 505-992-9904, dan@healthylivingspaces.com

ABOUT THE AUTHOR

As President of Healthy Living Spaces, Mr. Stih inspects residential and commercial buildings for mold and moisture. An aerospace engineer, Stih retired from Motorola and worked in construction before starting a mold inspection and testing company. He is a Council-Certified Microbial Consultant (CMC) and Council-Certified Indoor Environmental Consultant (CIEC), Board-awarded by the American Council for Accredited Certification (ACAC).

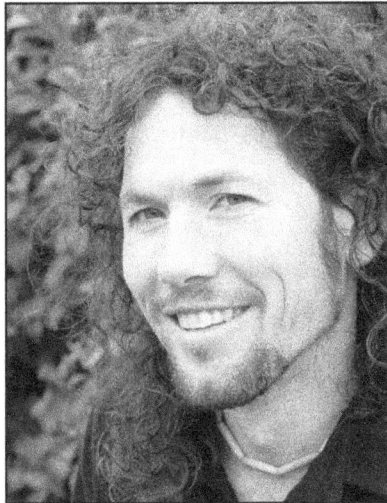

Stih studied Building Construction at Yavapai College with fieldwork building homes for Habitat for Humanity, holds a certificate, *Indoor Air Quality: Fungal Spore Identification* from the McCrone Research Institute, and partnered with Los Alamos National Laboratories to study and publish papers related to mold.

Author of the best seller, *Healthy Living Spaces: Top 10 Hazards Affecting Your Health*, Stih has been interviewed on over 100 radio and T.V. shows. Stih was hired by Dyson as an expert to provide consumers with tips on how to alleviate allergy symptoms and The National Kitchen and Bath Association (NKBA) to develop courses on selecting healthy building materials.

Stih is considered an expert witness in court and in depositions regarding evidence and facts related to mold.

Clients have included state and local governments, schools, hospitals, insurance companies, banks, hotels, shopping malls, police and fire stations and the homes of famous authors, actors, and sports celebrities.

Visit www.healthylivingspaces.com. If you are interested in learning how to look for mold (how to do a mold inspection) or how to test for mold, please goto www.academy.healthylivingspaces.com.

Stih lives in Santa Fe, New Mexico, travels the country to do inspections, is available for phone consultations and does expert witness testimony by phone appearance when required. For a list of speeches, papers and publications authored, media appearances and expert witness testimonies, please contact through the website and request a C.V.